Praise from experts
Adele Puhn's *The Car...*

"This user-friendly new book will give you effective tools to help you lose weight, lower cholesterol and blood pressure, and reduce your risks of breast cancer, heart disease, arthritis, and all other diseases of aging."
—Allan Warshowsky, M.D., founding diplomat of the American Board of Holistic Medicine

"This book is a brilliant expression of Adele's passion, insights, experience and talents. The connection between blood sugar regulation and wellness has long been her area of expertise and this book graciously provides theory, treatment and hope at a time when it is urgently needed."
—Sondra Kronberg, M.S., R.D., CDN, Co-Founder and Director, Eating Wellness Programs, New York

"Adele Puhn has changed my weight, my outlook, and my life."
—Marie Rao, president, Limited Brands

"Adele Puhn has topped herself! As wonderful as her past books were, she now takes losing weight and feeling great to a whole new level. This is a book for the way we live today."
—Phil Dusenberry, Chairman, BBDO North America

PENGUIN BOOKS

THE CARB-CAREFUL SOLUTION

Adele Puhn, M.S., C.N.S., a nutritional consultant with twenty-four years of experience, has a thriving practice in New York City and Long Island. She holds an M.S. in medical biology and clinical nutrition as well as the title Certified Nutrition Specialist from the American College of Nutrition. She is also a member of the board of the Professions of Dietetics and Nutrition in the State of New York. A popular speaker, lecturer, and author of several books including the *New York Times* bestseller *The 5-Day Miracle Diet*, Adele Puhn and her work have been featured in publications such as *Harper's Bazaar*, *The Wall Street Journal*, and *Cosmopolitan*. She lives in Manhasset, New York.

ALSO BY ADELE PUHN:

The 5-Day Miracle Diet
Healing from the Inside Out
The 5-Day Miracle Diet Companion
The Five Vital Secrets for a Healthy Life

THE
Carb-Careful
Solution

When Your Diet Doesn't
Work Anymore ...

ADELE PUHN, M.S., C.N.S.

Previously published as *The Midlife Miracle Diet*

Penguin Books

PENGUIN BOOKS

Published by the Penguin Group

Penguin Group (USA) Inc., 375 Hudson Street, New York, New York 10014, U.S.A.

Penguin Books Ltd, 80 Strand, London WC2R 0RL, England

Penguin Books Australia Ltd, 250 Camberwell Road, Camberwell,
  Victoria 3124, Australia

Penguin Books Canada Ltd, 10 Alcorn Avenue, Toronto, Ontario, Canada M4V 3B2

Penguin Books India (P) Ltd, 11 Community Centre, Panchsheel Park,
  New Delhi - 110 017, India

Penguin Books (N.Z.) Ltd, Cnr Rosedale and Airborne Roads, Albany,
  Auckland, New Zealand

Penguin Books (South Africa) (Pty) Ltd, 24 Sturdee Avenue, Rosebank,
  Johannesburg 2196, South Africa

Penguin Books Ltd, Registered Offices: 80 Strand, London WC2R 0RL, England

First published as *The Midlife Miracle Diet* in the United States of America
  by Viking Penguin, a member of Penguin Group (USA) Inc. 2003
Published as *The Carb-Careful Solution* in Penguin Books 2004

10 9 8 7 6 5 4 3 2 1

Copyright © Nutritional Industries, Inc., 2003
All rights reserved

THE LIBRARY OF CONGRESS HAS CATALOGED THE HARDCOVER EDITION AS FOLLOWS:
Puhn, Adele.
The midlife miracle diet : when your diet doesn't work anymore . . . / Adele Puhn.
p. cm.
Includes index.
ISBN 0-670-03168-2 (hc.)
ISBN 0 14 20.0376 X (pbk.)
1. Low-carbohydrate diet. I. Title.
RM237.73.P84 2003
613.2'83—dc21   2002069150

Printed in the United States of America
Designed by Susan Hood

FOR ARTHUR
who continues to show me that unwavering love
is the best food for the soul

ACKNOWLEDGMENTS

Throughout the writing of this book I have been lovingly surrounded by my interested and caring family, friends, and colleagues. My love for my children—Bonnee and Danny, Melissa and David, Alyson and Margot, and for their children: Charlotte, Lindsay, Jake, Zachary, Juliane, and Baby Noah—provided powerful inspiration to write about what may be a part of their genetic blueprint. I am forever grateful to the many friends who offered not only encouragement, but also contributed each in their own special way. Nutritionist Sondra Kronberg took time out of her impossibly busy schedule to review and discuss the shaping of the manuscript. Margery Weinroth and Eleanor Dubin were invaluable offering both encourgement and ideas after reading the early, difficult stages of the manuscript. I was pleased to have nutritionist Joy Suskin offer special insights, based on her familiarity with both my programs and my philosophy. Thanks and deep appreciation to those people who were there, supplying constant interest and loving support as kindling for the creative fires: Donna Gelman, Diana and Stanley Langer, Ellie Rothschild, Susan Hans, Maxine Pines, Sydelle Prince, Marty, Mary, and Jared Green, and certainly not the least—Uncle Hank and Aunt Helen.

Acknowledgments

As always, without my clients there could be no book. I want to thank them all for being actively involved and supportive of my ongoing work. Their willing participation and passionate quest for a better life has been the motivation to create this program.

Special thanks to my agent, Wendy Weil, who was excited, as always, to hear my new ideas while offering her sage advice and constant support. I am particularly grateful to my collaborator, Billie Fitzpatrick, whose considerable talent, organizational skills, and calm presence were instrumental in the creation of this book. The wonderful staff at Viking has my deep appreciation, especially my publisher, Clare Ferraro, who was not only supportive and enthusiastic but also understood my work in a very special and important way. Many thanks go to my editor, Janet Goldstein, for trusting me to go forward with the manuscript, developing it as I imagined it would be. The publicist Cindy Hamel and art director Roseanne Serra, thank you for your unique and critical contributions to the success of this book.

I want to thank Jeffrey Bland for disseminating his groundbreaking research in his annual seminars that allowed so many health practitioners to enhance and extend the quality of life for their clients. Adam Banning placed himself, and his vast resources of nutrient research, at my disposal, applying his considerable knowledge to help me work out some of the knottier issues of formulating a supplement program that could be effective in this book. I would also like to extend my appreciation to Metagenics Inc. for making its vast research archives available and for allowing the adaptation of its excellent illustration of cellular blood sugar metabolism. Dr. Alan Warshowsky, gynecologist extraordinaire, offered critical technical advice after reading the manuscript. His input has been especially valuable.

Finally, I want to give my deepest thanks to my husband, Arthur, for his loving interest and hard work. He has remained, as always, my soul mate, offering his love, support, and advice when most needed. His steadfast belief that one should always reach for the stars has encouraged me to stretch beyond any imagined limits.

Note to Readers

The advice, information, and guidelines presented in this book are not intended to replace professional medical advice. Any reader—especially one with a preexisting medical condition—should consult first with a qualified health-care practitioner before starting this program. If you are currently taking medication for type 2 diabetes, high blood pressure, or for any other condition, consult your physician before taking any supplements. While the author has attempted to ensure that the information presented is accurate up to the time of publication, medical knowledge is constantly evolving and ongoing research may lead to changes in some of the concepts presented in this book.

The case histories in this book are based on actual clients; however, in all cases, names and identifying characteristics have been changed.

CONTENTS

Contents

INTRODUCTION

In 1995 my career as a nutritionist changed completely. I went from being a one-on-one nutrition counselor and lecturer to author of *The 5-Day Miracle Diet*. Adding this dimension to my work opened up my world: I was able to share my approach to nutrition with thousands more people both in print and on television and radio. This opportunity was exciting and rewarding beyond my wildest dreams not only because I was suddenly able to reach a much wider audience but also because the responses to my work have continued to inspire my passion for finding solutions for optimal health.

In my first book I was able to tell the story of my personal odyssey that led me to the discovery that putting an end to carbohydrate craving is the key to achieving balanced blood sugar control. I was overwhelmed by the response to *The 5-Day Miracle Diet*. This book showed that there is an enormous population of people who, like me, had been struggling to control their carbohydrate cravings. Thankfully, it provided a solution that gave most of these people back their lives. Readers from all over the world shared their similar struggles and their gratitude for hearing my story, and their letters and calls still warm my heart. That was my first miracle.

As a nutritionist I have been passionate about blood sugar control for years, and my work with thousands of men and women has enabled me to study the intricacies of body chemistry up close and personal. Now, more than ever, I have seen the impact of how life is fueled by too much or too little blood sugar and how what we eat affects how we experience our lives. I know this for sure: A well-fed, well-nourished body can allow someone to live a healthy, vibrant life.

When I developed the 5-Day Diet, it was a weight-loss program, and while it was a healthy way to lose weight, I was not focused on overall health. In the intervening years, I have had a chance to both broaden and sharpen my focus as I've researched and evaluated the interplay between carbohydrates, insulin, and blood sugar control and how the interaction of these three components impacts the body's health. This close scrutiny has paid off: As I examined the intricacies of the relationship between carbohydrate cravings (the result of blood sugar control gone awry) and insulin function, I began to observe a very serious disorder of metabolism, which I came to call the Metabolic Mix-Up, whose most specific cause is insulin resistance.

Though basic blood sugar control still works beautifully for many people, I have seen that there is still a large group of people who, because of their Metabolic Mix-Up, need another level of control to curb these cravings and balance their blood sugar. And I'm part of this group! I always wondered why if I upset my blood sugar balance even slightly, I would soon be eating a whole box of cookies instead of just one or two to satisfy my craving. Like the most reactive clients in my office, I have always had to work harder at controlling my blood sugar. Why? Because this higher degree of sensitivity to carbs, for some of my clients as well as myself, too often accompanied a series of conditions such as high blood pressure, high cholesterol, high triglycerides, a tendency to high blood sugar, exhaustion, and overall aches and pains. Because this cluster of serious conditions would occur and reoccur in my most carbohydrate-connected and insulin-resistant clients, I began to wonder if this was yet a more dangerous level of reactions orchestrated by blood sugar that was out of control.

Alarmingly, this Metabolic Mix-Up is so common that most people tend to disregard the signs and not take them seriously. The many people streaming through my office come in all shapes and sizes: They are children and adolescents, busy thirty-five-year olds, fast-aging baby boomers in their fifties, and people in their seventies. Too many have begun to develop high blood pressure and high cholesterol, with type 2 diabetes a frequent issue in their families. They are some of the millions who have always wanted to lose those ten or fifteen extra pounds, who crave carbohydrates, who have a chronic sweet tooth, who lose weight and gain it right back. Sound at all familiar? They are seemingly healthy men and women in their thirties and forties and fifties who would never dream that they have a metabolic disorder so serious that it can develop into diabetes, heart disease, and the risk of stroke.

Just as my clients were instrumental in my writing of *The 5-Day Miracle Diet,* insisting that I spread the word, many of the women and men with whom I work in my practice encouraged me to share their experiences with my new dietary program, the Carb-Careful Solution. Before doing the program, these men and women had no idea that the foods they were eating could impact so dramatically on their daily existence, and they wanted others outside of my office to know. So grateful for their new lease on life, they wanted me to share this information so you too can discover the key to a richer quality of life.

Welcome to my office. Pull up a chair and let the adventure begin, an adventure that can save your life.

PART ONE

Your Body's Chemistry

———— ∞∞ ————

CHAPTER 1

Meet Your Metabolic Mix-Up

STOPPING DISEASE IN ITS TRACKS

I don't usually resort to scare tactics to encourage people to get healthy; however, in this case the news is so frightening and significant that I feel it is my responsibility to spread the word.

Over the past several years I have listened to client after client describe the same set of problems—a chronic lack of energy, high blood pressure, high cholesterol, and stubborn overweight that won't budge. I became more and more concerned. What was going on? All of these symptoms are the same as those that accompany type 2 diabetes. And recently, the mainstream media has delivered a blitz of information about a growing diabetes epidemic in America—just one of several health conditions that can be addressed by the Carb-Careful Solution!

Consider some of the headlines: *Newsweek* announced "An American Epidemic: Diabetes" and *The New York Times* warns "Diabetes as Looking Epidemic." An even more recent *New York Times* article entitled "As Diabetes Strikes Younger, Children Get Lessons in Defense" points out the increase in the occurrence of diabetes type 2 cases—this time in children. The media has also begun to highlight our casual disregard for other life-threatening diseases. Another *New York Times* article entitled "A Devastating

Lack of Awareness: Why Women Don't Believe Heart Disease, Their No. 1 Killer, Really Affects Them" is self-explanatory.

Working on the front lines of nutrition, I am not surprised by this increase in diabetes and many people's lack of awareness of the state of their overall health. I see a direct link between these diseases and a disorder of metabolism every day in my office, and I am concerned, very concerned. What concerns me most is that many people—millions in fact—are walking around like accidents waiting to happen, completely unaware that they have already developed what I call the Metabolic Mix-Up.

This disorder of metabolism was first identified as Syndrome X by Dr. George Reaven of Stanford University when he discovered the link between insulin resistance and serious disease, including type 2 diabetes and heart disease. The syndrome is characterized by six traits: insulin resistance, glucose intolerance, abnormally high insulin levels, high triglycerides, low high-density lipoprotein (the *good* cholesterol), and hypertension.

I soon was able to see that many of my clients were actually suffering from symptoms of this Metabolic Mix-Up, a disorder of metabolism so profound, so life impacting that it literally controls our body chemistry and can shorten our lives unless we stop it. I became determined to find not only a solution but also the reason behind this metabolic disorder that has become so prevalent. *The Carb-Careful Solution* is the result of my search for these answers.

THE MENACING METABOLIC MIX-UP

Let me ask you a few questions:

1. Do you attend cultural events and become more annoyed and distracted by the noise than uplifted by the performance?
2. Have your blood pressure and cholesterol climbed every year?
3. Do you wake up in the morning, already sighing as the alarm tries to jump-start you?

4. Have you recently put on weight around your middle that you are unable to shed?
5. Do new challenges at work make you feel overwhelmed instead of creative?
6. Does planning a last-minute pleasure trip become a nightmare?
7. Do you feel so lethargic that you can barely last through your son's baseball game?
8. Has your doctor warned you to lose some weight because your blood sugar is testing too high?
9. At the end of most days does your bed seem the only place you want to be?
10. Do you feel older than your age?
11. Are you so exhausted after getting through the work week that by Friday, you can't even imagine going out for the evening?

If you answered yes to several of these questions, then you more than likely have the Metabolic Mix-Up. This disorder works so devilishly behind the curtain of your life that you may not even know you are developing serious symptoms. It could be the player behind your frequent headaches, malaise, and your recent inability to lose weight. It could also be the cause of your recent increase in blood pressure and cholesterol. The Metabolic Mix-Up is so powerful, so crafty, that it can impact on your minute-to-minute life.

Men and women with the mix-up feel just this way: They can get through the week, but that's about it. They have no energy left to enjoy life. In fact they can't even begin to imagine how they *should* feel. They have literally become hostages of their own bodies, unable to connect to their health potential.

We are not surprised when we develop high blood pressure and high cholesterol; after all, these are two very common ailments that don't make us think twice. We accept them as natural by-products of aging. They certainly don't sound off alarm bells, but they should. This cluster of symptoms may not look alarming at first glance, but think about this: They are connected to the three most common causes of death in this country—heart disease, stroke, and type 2 diabetes.

You may not yet have high blood pressure or high cholesterol, but you might just have the genetic wiring or lifestyle habits that lead directly to the Metabolic Mix-Up. Make no mistake: This is not an excessive warning. The millions of people who are fast developing type 2 diabetes and other degenerative diseases are just like the men and women who arrive at my doorstep, bringing with them all the signs that the Metabolic Mix-Up is at play.

TYPE 1 OR TYPE 2? THERE IS A DIFFERENCE

There are two major types of diabetes, and insulin is the protagonist in both diseases. The majority (about 90 percent of cases) of people who have diabetes have type 2 diabetes, which can be caused by insulin resistance: the cell's inability to use or let insulin into the cell to convert the food we eat into cellular energy. Type 1 diabetes (formerly called juvenile diabetes or insulin-dependent diabetes) accounts for only 10 percent of diabetes cases and usually appears in children. Type 1 diabetes is caused by the attack of the immune system on the cells in the pancreas that produce insulin, resulting in an inability to produce insulin. Unlike type 2 diabetics (or noninsulin-dependent diabetics), type 1 diabetics must take insulin injections for survival. However, most type 2 diabetics do not need to take insulin, and in many cases, taking insulin would only aggravate and worsen their condition.

The Metabolic Mix-Up can be so devastating that it has also been linked to some cancers. It's already been shown that women with high insulin levels who are receiving standard therapy for breast cancer were eight times more likely to experience cancer recurrence and die of the disease than were patients with normal insulin levels. I have considered the possibility of a link between this disorder of metabolism and cancer for a while and have wondered whether the high rates of breast cancer in pockets of the northeast could be linked not only to the high level of contaminants in the water and possible electromagnetic fields, as well as other environmental factors, but also to the high-carb, low-fat, pasta-is-king diet that began in the late 1970s. Remember when we first started hearing about a low-fat diet? With that revolution came pasta. I saw this latest approach overtake the American conscience. Given the green light, thousands of weight-conscious women and men began eating pasta and other starchy carbohydrates with abandon, believing that by simply staying away from fat they would be slimmer and healthier. Wanting to look good, lose weight, and enhance their health, they embraced a way of eating that in fact challenged their ability to process insulin, the hormonal instrument that metabolizes carbohydrates.

The 1970s and 1980s also saw vegetarianism gaining more attention as a way of life, not just moralistically but because people had suddenly become more interested in eating better and leaving behind the American meat-and-potatoes legacy. However, each of us has a biochemical individuality. For some, vegetarian eating is an improvement and a benefit for their health. But for others, those of us with the Metabolic Mix-Up, it's not okay. In fact, it's lethal.

It wasn't until fourteen years ago, after I was diagnosed with breast cancer and was recovering from a lumpectomy that I began to understand that something was not working. As you can imagine, I was shocked that I could get this disease. After all, I was a vegetarian who meditated, jogged, ate organic food, and drank gallons of bottled water. What had happened to my body? Fortunately, the lumpectomy was successful and I was safely in remission. But I had learned a very hard, very scary lesson.

In my search to understand, I began to suspect that something else was working behind the scenes of my health, something I had not known or thought about. During the sensitive recuperation period, as I worked hard to restore my health and regain my strength, I had switched from an ovo-lacto-vegetarian diet to a macrobiotic diet, hoping to benefit from its special healing qualities. Yet after only ten days of following the macrobiotic diet, composed of 80 percent grains and beans (i.e., carbohydrates), I gained ten very puffy pounds. Gone was my sculpted body of which I had been so proud! My small waist (always my best feature) was no more as I began to take on an apple shape. Feeling very fatigued, I found myself craving sugar wildly, plotting to get my favorite cookies at eight o'clock in the morning. After years of freedom from my sugar addiction, I was feeling needier, more connected to cravings than ever. I tried to sort out what was happening to my body and began to feel that my reaction had to be connected to my increased intake of carbohydrates. That was all that had changed in my diet. I had been a vegetarian—this is true—but I had been a vegetarian who ate lots of tofu, vegetables, and small amounts of eggs, beans, and grains. Stunned by my instant reactiveness to the major increase in grains and beans, I wanted to understand what was going on.

When I followed the trail, it led me right back to where my reactiveness to carbohydrates had begun in the first place.

MY PARENTS CAME FIRST

As a Sugar Baby, I was both born to my parents and formed by them. And in their overreliance on bread *with* dinner and dessert *after* dinner, they set the stage not only for their own disordered metabolism but mine as well. Their attachment to sweets and starches not only left them in that familiar state of exhaustion and lethargy but it also had another significant effect: It made a huge impression on me as a child. I not only craved sugar (their constant companion) but as I grew older I also craved a solution to my parents' obvious distress. Through my child's wide eyes, they seemed unable to relax and enjoy themselves, even after a long week of working hard. My parents were also reliant on medications to treat their high blood pressure and cholesterol and to ease their aches and pains. Like a cozy hearth, the medicine chest in my parents' bathroom was central to our lives, a familiar gathering place where the family could feel its common bond. At any one time, I could open the door and see an array of different sized bottles and containers with all sorts of medications—for high blood pressure, high cholesterol, high triglycerides, tranquilizers, insulin, and aspirin—all the popular fixings to treat their unnamed Metabolic Mix-Up!

Of course, as a child I had little idea of what these magical bottles contained or what they were for. It's only now, years later, that I wonder if this medication really warmed their hearts or merely kept their bodies functioning? They would go to the doctor complaining of shortness of breath, fatigue, or headaches, and the doctor would write them the recommended prescription, once again sending them down the path that could not lead to recovery. This was the way it was done and overdone—the standard approach—at the time. Now I know that my parents and their friends depended on these mysterious little glass containers and the magic potions inside as a way to manage all their physical and emotional problems. They didn't know (nor did their doctors nor anyone else in the health field) that what was causing their high cholesterol and out-of-control blood pressure, as well as their malaise, fatigue, and overweight were the very real side effects of their ordinary but destructive eating habits and sedentary lifestyles. They also didn't know that what was behind this cluster of conditions was the very destructive side effects of their insulin resistance.

Sadly, I did not connect the dots of my parents' lives soon enough. By his mature middle years, my father had full-blown type 2 diabetes that had to be treated with insulin injections, while my mother's days were filled with an ongoing struggle to lose weight and manage her hypertension. They continued to eat the sweets and starches that fed their out-of-control chemistry, while the increasing medications merely eased some of the pain but didn't address the problem.

Yet I know that my vision of the two of them seeking answers but finding none fueled my lifelong obsession to understand the relationship between eating habits and health. And though I was not able to help my parents tame their Metabolic Mix-Up, I can and do help thousands of the women and men who come to see me in my office and read my books, and now I want to help you and those you love.

MEDICATIONS CAN HAVE SIDE EFFECTS

Controlling the Metabolic Mix-Up can help to control disorders that create the need for powerful drugs.

THE SUGAR CONNECTION

My own story and that of my parents highlights an important feature of the Metabolic Mix-Up: a strong and passionate friendship with starchy foods and sweets. Do you see yourself in the questions below? How many would you answer yes to?

1. Is your diet comprised mostly of white flour and mushy, starchy foods?
2. Do you rely on diet soda or tea drinks as your main source of fluids?
3. Do you often meet your friends for a before-dinner drink, followed by another one or two after dinner?
4. Is the only green food on your plate or in your refrigerator a few grapes?
5. Are your four main food groups bread, bread, bread, and more bread?
6. Is it impossible for you to spend an evening that doesn't include a snack?

7. Do you never leave home without a fistful of hard candies or gum?
8. Is pasta your manna from heaven?

If you answered yes to two or more of the above questions, then more than likely you fall into that familiar group that I call Sugar Babies, of which I am a starring member. These dietary tendencies are just a few of the signs that you may have the chemistry that misfires in the presence of sugar and other carbohydrates. This misfiring can cause powerful food connections and these cravings are one of the clearest indications that the Metabolic Mix-Up may be stamped into your genes. Sugar Babies from Sugar Baby Land, there are so many of us, whether from years of relying on starches and sugars as our major source of food or from some other genetic twist of fate.

But you don't have to awaken these sleeping genes. Some Europeans, specifically those people who live on or near the Mediterranean, don't demonstrate Sugar Baby characteristics. They grow up eating a diet totally different from the typical American fare. Instead of our meat and potatoes, they eat a lot of fish, raw and cooked vegetables, and fruit. The result? This Mediterranean training does not awaken or reinforce reactive chemistry.

Who said life was fair?

Essentially, if you have a diet that is high in sugar and carbs and you are already predisposed to be sensitive to them, then you are unwittingly reinforcing your insulin resistance.

LET THE CARB-CAREFUL SOLUTION BE YOUR ANSWER

Have you ever heard of the French expression joie de vivre? To me, it captures everything remarkable about being alive: living life with passion, resolve, clarity of mind, a full heart, and a body brimming with energy and health. The Carb-Careful Solution not only leads you away from the perils of disease, it leads you toward a life filled with joie de vivre—joy in living!

Like many of my clients, you may be wondering if there is some kind of magic pill, a silver bullet, that will heal all your ills and make you feel great both inside and out. And even though this is not an instant cure, it can be magic. Find out for yourself. All you have to do is follow the four-step program that follows.

The Carb-Careful Solution is the program I've developed for the millions of women and men who love carbohydrates and don't want to see them disappear from their lives. If you, like me, have this Metabolic Mix-Up, there is great news: on the Carb-Careful Solution, you don't have to worry about cutting your wonderful carbohydrates out of your life forever. Instead, you simply need to learn how and when to eat them.

The men and women in my practice are of varying ages and varying backgrounds. Some are businessmen and -women ready to retire, others have returned home to raise a family, and still others are just starting out in the fashion industry, work at a media company, manage a retail shop, or work on Wall Street. My clients represent an enormous range of people from busy New Yorkers to a woman who lives in a forest outside of Yosemite National Park. Many of these men and women were referred to me by their doctors for nutritional counseling because they needed more than medicine to help treat their high blood pressure, high cholesterol, and aches and pains. Some people came to see me wanting to lose five to ten pounds; others arrived seriously overweight, with at least one hundred pounds to lose. Still others came worried about their apparent need to go on medication for their cholesterol or high blood pressure. But very few of them knew to come because they have a disorder of metabolism that can lead to type 2 diabetes, stroke, or breast cancer.

CAPTURE THE SPIRIT OF JOIE DE VIVRE

The essence of joie de vivre is living life to its fullest—in energy, clarity of mind, and strength of purpose. When you discover your own joie de vivre, you will wake with a song in your heart and a smile on your face.

You are reading this book so that you can learn once and for all how to take care of yourself so that you too enjoy the best life possible. In four steps you will curb habits that impact your reactive chemistry and learn how to tame the main cause of the Metabolic Mix-Up—your insulin resistance—by defusing your carbohydrate reactions, balancing your blood sugar, and enhancing your insulin function. You can not only reprogram your body's metabolic system so that it works more efficiently to use carbohydrates (the body and brain's main source of energy), but you will also burn fat and strengthen your immune system. In short, you will control the chemistry that has been controlling you.

As a practitioner, I knew that I had to design the Carb-Careful Solution so that it would be doable and livable so that you can easily *own* the diet and no longer think twice about eating in this new way. I wanted it to become as natural to you as getting up in the morning and taking a shower, getting in your car and driving to work, or hugging your child before he lies down to sleep at night.

THE CARB-CAREFUL SOLUTION IS A WAY OF LIFE

Even though this program is called a diet, it's more a way of life. There is no deprivation, no great restriction of foods. You can eat plentifully and from an array of wonderful foods.

You can pack this program with you as you travel, go to work, and dine in restaurants. The difference between success and failure is as simple as pairing your apple with some almonds for a snack or learning to keep bananas and berries out of your morning menu. You'll no longer create your schedule based on what you *can't* do because you're too sick, too tired, too overweight, or too frustrated. You'll soon be chasing after yourself as you join that chorus group you always wanted to, take that trip to Paris you and your husband have always dreamed about, make love with your partner . . . twice in the same night.

Joan came to see me with the classic signs of the Metabolic Mix-Up: Her blood pressure and LDL cholesterol had soared, she had become unable to shed a nagging fifteen pounds, which seemed permanently wrapped around what used to be her waist. She also felt demoralized by an allover malaise that was making her depressed and anxious. After just a few weeks on the Carb-Careful Solution, Joan not only lost ten pounds but she had also lost all her muscle fatigue as well. "I am so thrilled with this program. This is so darn good. I never felt better. I'm never going to be a sick, fat, tired person again. I've got the answer, and I am so grateful. You are a new friend in my life!" Joan is so happy with her new approach to life that she even goes on the Web describing how much her life has changed for the better. She still finds it incredible that she has actually eliminated the chemistry that was going to lead to life-threatening conditions.

I am passionate about wanting to help all of you, convince you to change your habits so that you don't walk in my parents' footsteps. When you direct your body to function better, you will *feel* remarkably better. You will feel better in your mind and in your heart. Your days will become more enjoyable, you will feel more energetic and passionate about life again. You will get in touch with that joie de vivre that makes you want to call an old friend, start a new book, or run up the side of a mountain. As one of my clients, Nicole, a forty-two-year-old fashion designer, said to me recently, "I finally feel fine in my life. I've never felt normal before. My cholesterol was always high. And I was tired of everyone around me being so thin—you know how models eat very low fat all the time. I was sure they didn't have any cholesterol problems. But now that I'm on the diet, I actually feel happy. I only expected to change some medical problems, not get a whole new life. I'm losing weight and can handle stress so much better and my cholesterol readings are perfect. As a matter of fact, I am the only one in my family who has normal cholesterol." Her newfound joy in living was ringing in her voice.

I am fortunate to be able to be part of such happy transformations. Again and again, I have been able to see the power that taking care of yourself can have on your being.

Just as we have redefined our understanding of aging by distinguishing between biological and chronological age, so too should we redefine the middle part of our life span. Instead of thinking of midlife as the step before old age, I suggest we approach this stage of life as the time to appreciate all that we have accomplished—and with the Carb-Careful Solution, one of our major accomplishments will be a prolonged sense of vitality that we normally reserve for youth. So here's to redefining your midlife by making it the *best* time in your life!

CHAPTER 2

What's Behind Your Metabolic Mix-Up?

DON'T SAY OKAY TO FEELING MEDIOCRE

In my twenty-two years of nutritional counseling, helping men and women to get healthy and stay healthy, I have been amazed at how many don't *really* know how well they can feel; they don't realize that they possess the power to *create* good health. One of my clients just learned this powerful lesson. For years, at the end of the day, she would feel so exhausted, she would barely be able to speak on the phone. She'd say this was because she got up at 6:00 A.M. and had a full day. I finally convinced her that she was not supposed to feel like this. I said to her, "Why have you allowed yourself to accept your high blood pressure and high cholesterol? You don't have to feel this way!" She responded, "But I'm taking my medications and following the low-fat and low-sodium diet that I'm supposed to." I told her she needed to learn more, to ask for more, to work toward getting what should be hers—the best quality of life possible.

What we are used to thinking of as normal is very far from how we *should* feel. What we are used to thinking of as normal is really mediocre, and as a result, many people are living lives of mediocre health, nowhere near the full potential that is in their reach. But they also don't have anything to compare their lives to, no gauge for understanding that they are not in optimal health and have never felt vibrant. And as a result, by default, they just accept mediocrity.

ARE YOU LIVING LIFE AT HALF-MAST?

Do you get up in the morning, go to work, push through until evening only by having a little pick-me-up as a reward for getting through the day? If so, then you might be living life at half-mast.

Would you believe me if I said that most of you live life at half-mast, so accustomed to feeling mediocre or "just okay" that you are not able even to imagine what it feels like to be in great health? Recently, Connie, a forty-four-year-old woman, came to me completely fed up with her life. She'd gotten to the point where she felt so tired and lethargic all the time that she was convinced that she had fibromyalgia and chronic fatigue, not to mention a serious conviction that her thyroid was totally at fault. Like many of you, Connie is a highly able, competent, and accomplished woman who is doing well at her job and raising her children, but at great cost: She had barely enough energy to enjoy the rest of her life. But even sadder than this forfeit of potential is the fact that she had no clue that she didn't have to feel this way. That is the impact of the Metabolic Mix-Up. It depletes your life of energy and you don't even realize it.

THE WAY YOU SHOULD FEEL

- You wake up in the morning feeling refreshed; you may need an alarm but it's no great punishment to get out of bed.
- You feel calm and comfortable as you face the day.
- You have an I-can-do mentality.
- You experience a vibrant store of energy throughout your daily activities.
- You appreciate the end of your day instead of feeling devastated and worn out.

THE CHEMISTRY CONNECTION

I have seen the transformation again and again: When clients eat right, they are happy and joyful. They do what they need to do with energy, verve, and confidence. But when they don't eat right, eat too many carbohydrates, or don't get enough exercise, they lose their life force and their I-can-do attitude that empowers them to accomplish whatever they want to do. This crucial difference is the most simple, immediate result of having the Metabolic Mix-Up. And how you eat is directly related to controlling your body chemistry. For those of us with the Metabolic Mix-Up, we are even more sensitive to the chemical swings within the body.

Your chemistry dictates how your body operates. In the same way that an operating system allows a computer to run a certain program, your body chemistry (your operating system) tells you how to feel. Therefore when your chemistry is set up to feel mediocre, either by genetic destiny or in reaction to your lifestyle, you'll feel mediocre. But if you take control of your chemistry and reprogram it to feel great, you will feel great. And with feeling great comes the added, incomparable bonus of avoiding disease and premature aging.

CONTROL YOUR CHEMISTRY SO IT DOESN'T CONTROL YOU

Most people want to resist the idea that their daily fusilli or pizza fix is really a craving. They'd rather call it a habit, a temptation, or more often they will assault their lack of willpower. No, it is very simply a craving and a craving is the creator of habit. So many people defend against cravings by explaining that their cookies or chips at night are just a habit, that they always have done this. While there is some reality to all of this, there is also chemistry. Chemistry that sets up a craving so powerful that it convinces you it's your idea. By and large, once you have redirected your chemistry, you will feel so free that you'll be able to detach easily from the heady games that food has played on you for years.

At the heart of your chemistry is blood sugar control. Quite simply, if you are not eating right you are affecting your chemistry: You will either be in high blood sugar or low blood sugar—somewhere on the pendulum that keeps swinging, unless you anchor your chemistry and lock it into place. When your blood sugar is too low or too high, you can feel depressed, anxious, and restless. You are vulnerable to a wide range of mood swings. But once your blood sugar is in balance, the way you feel—your emotional state of being—translates into a joy for living.

This connection between chemistry and how you feel became more real than ever before in the aftermath of the terrible attack on the World Trade Center in New York City. In the days and weeks that followed this event, people in my practice tended to fall into two groups: Either they had no appetite and couldn't even think about food, or they were eating everything in sight. But for either camp, I gave the same instructions: They had to deliver food to their bodies as a source of nourishment—physically, mentally, emotionally, and spiritually—in order to calm themselves enough to function and cope.

Think about this: Your brain is 3 percent of your body weight, but it uses 20 percent of the energy from your food. Your brain also requires a constant replenishment of this energy because it can't store any, and it is therefore critically important to keep your blood sugar in balance. As soon as you slip, your brain is affected. So if you're not eating or you're eating the wrong things, you are going to feel more stressed, more tired, more lethargic. You're going to be suffering more anxiety and depression, making you less able to cope and focus. You have to take care of yourself: You have to take care of that brain that is going to tell you how to feel.

And though this tragedy made it even more crucial to control our chemistry, we need to listen to this mantra every day of our lives. If you talk to your chemistry, giving it the right messages, then you will not only feel much better in your life, you will discover your true potential for feeling good—physically, emotionally, and mentally. Beth, the mother of a special needs child, discovered the rewards of controlling her chemistry. She explained, "The difference in how I feel is so incredible. I am so much more hopeful about my son. I could never talk myself into a positive attitude. Now, without trying, I just feel confident that I can help him. And you know what else—I am enjoying his company so much more. I feel like my whole life changed when I changed my daily menus." This is the power of the chemistry connection.

The first step you must take is to take responsibility and see what condition your body is really in. The program you are about to embark upon does just that: It begins by showing you how to assess your health and ends by controlling your chemistry so it doesn't control you. By controlling your chemistry, you can avoid the perils of disease and no longer live life at half-mast. Discovering your potential for stopping the inevitability of disease and learning how to live fully is all about learning how to take care of yourself. You need to discover how well you can feel. Once you get yourself into good chemistry, you too will feel uplifted. Not only will life's stresses seem much more manageable, but you will also discover a joie de vivre—a joy in living that in the past escaped you.

THE INS AND OUTS OF INSULIN

The first step to taming your Metabolic Mix-Up is by controlling your chemistry, and this means controlling insulin. Throughout the Carb-Careful Solution, you are going to hear insulin named again and again as being at the root of many diseases, not only diabetes. This vital hormone is at the heart of the Metabolic Mix-Up.

Like most things in life, insulin has both positive and negative qualities. When it's behaving well, your body hums: You eat a meal and your pancreas responds by releasing insulin to carry the glucose into the cell for energy. It's insulin's job to ensure your body's proper metabolism.

But when insulin misbehaves and either can't get into cells or is overproduced, or both, then it perpetuates a number of metabolic reactions that lead to serious, life-threatening diseases. Almost without exception, if there is not some sort of equalizing factor like a change in diet, exercise, or use of supplements, this disruption in your metabolism can result in a very poor quality of life or an early death.

How does insulin work? Just imagine that insulin is a train whose cargo is glucose and whose destination is the body's cells that rely on delivery of energy. When the insulin train is functioning properly, the cell opens its door to the glucose transport and your body receives its necessary delivery of energy. However, when insulin cannot penetrate the cell wall (as is the case when you have the Metabolic Mix-Up), the fuel is not delivered. Without this fuel, the body has no energy.

Healthy Insulin

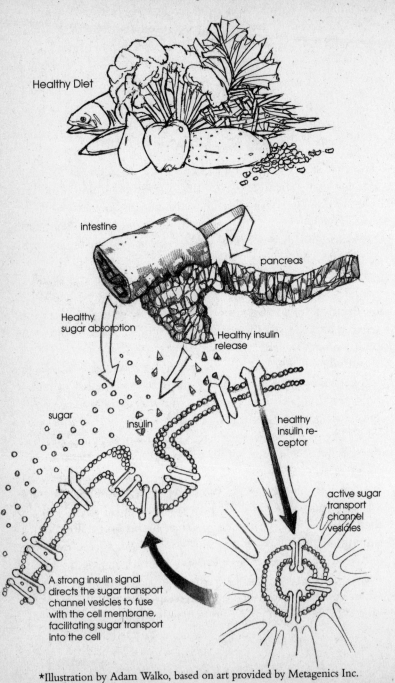

Healthy Diet

intestine

pancreas

Healthy sugar absorption

Healthy insulin release

sugar

insulin

healthy insulin re-ceptor

active sugar transport channel vesicles

A strong insulin signal directs the sugar transport channel vesicles to fuse with the cell membrane, facilitating sugar transport into the cell

*Illustration by Adam Walko, based on art provided by Metagenics Inc.

Unhealthy Insulin

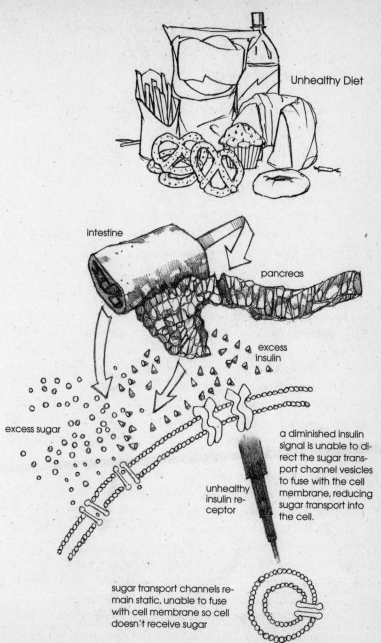

Unhealthy Diet

intestine

pancreas

excess insulin

excess sugar

a diminished insulin signal is unable to direct the sugar transport channel vesicles to fuse with the cell membrane, reducing sugar transport into the cell.

unhealthy insulin receptor

sugar transport channels remain static, unable to fuse with cell membrane so cell doesn't receive sugar

static sugar transport vesicle

YOUR CHEMISTRY GONE AWRY

This is what the impetuous cycle of insulin resistance looks like for those of us with the Metabolic Mix-Up:

- When we eat carbohydrates our cells don't respond to the insulin knocking on the door.
- Our body responds by producing more insulin in an attempt to force entry into cells.
- Only the smallest amount of insulin can penetrate our cells in order to deliver the food for energy.
- We're left feeling even more cravings, more lethargic, and to add insult to injury, the roaming insulin is quickly signaling the body to store fat.

This dysfunction in insulin is called insulin resistance. Essentially, insulin resistance is an inability (or weak ability) of the receptor cell's acceptance of insulin. Insulin resistance means that the cell cannot receive the insulin necessary to deliver the glucose—the energy necessary for life. There are several possible causes for insulin resistance, including an inherited tendency toward this chemical dysfunction, a reaction to a lifetime pattern of eating foods high in fat, starch, and sugar, and a lack of exercise.

Insulin resistance can eventually result in *hyperinsulinemia*—an overproduction of insulin. With the Metabolic Mix-Up, these two conditions create a catch-22 pattern that is played and replayed in the body as the insulin tries, again and again, to penetrate the cell. At the level of the cell, insulin resistance is an inability of the insulin receptor to direct the sugar transport channel vesicles to fuse with the cell membrane. When this fusion does not occur, the nucleus of the cell does not receive the sugar. When the insulin cannot get into the cells, the cells can't process the food you eat, specifically the carbohydrates, to deliver energy. You're left feeling tired, lethargic, and lacking in vitality. Remember high school biology and the word *homeostasis,* the balance necessary for life? Insulin is not supposed to remain in the blood stream. In an attempt to restore the necessary balance, however misguided, the circulating insulin taps you on the shoulder and says, "Excuse me, I have nothing to do. You better eat more carbohydrates so that I can be busy." But look out! In an attempt to force entry into the cell, more insulin is produced, feeding into a continuing, uncontrollable craving that makes you want and need to eat more and more carbohydrates. This ongoing intake of carbohydrates encourages the body to continue to overproduce insulin—an action that was already in motion. You now have become hyperinsulinemic and have way too much insulin circulating. Hyperinsulinemia is the body's answer to the problem of trying to get the insulin into the cell. But as a result your body will continue to produce more and more insulin under the misguided notion that more is better, reinforcing its stubborn will to get into the cell, but no doors will swing open. With increased force, the insulin train bangs on the cell's wall but only a small amount may manage to get through.

But what about the rest? What about homeostasis? Since insulin is a storage hormone, the excess insulin must take the remaining glucose, unable to be used for energy, and store it as fat. As a part of this chemical blueprint the insulin calls for the release of the enzyme lipoprotein lipase that directs the body to store fat. This dangerous fat buildup is what contributes to hardening of the arteries, high cholesterol, high blood pressure, high triglycerides, obesity, and even greater insulin resistance. Welcome to the land of the Metabolic Mix-Up.

This never-ending cycle is why you are so accustomed to feeling tired. You think there is nothing unusual about this feeling. Everybody around you is tired. But isn't it a relief to know there is actually a reason besides staying up too late, a reason that makes you more exhausted than you should be? But how can you know? What gauge do you have to measure how vital you should be? Should? Yes, should be. You were designed to go through the days and hours and minutes feeling wonderful, not just okay.

WEAR AND TEAR THAT CAN DAMAGE YOUR LIFE

Unchecked, insulin resistance challenges your body's ability to protect itself from illness and the normal stresses of the environment. Immune disorders such as lupus and chronic fatigue can be the result of this wear and tear. Your overreactive chemistry and the strain of living in overdrive depletes your body. You end up living on the edge, a target for disaster.

VANQUISHING THE INSULIN INSULT

For so many years this single major problem, insulin resistance, remained a mystery. Because of its subtle nature, too many people, including my parents, followed orders (orders based on the only information available) and took medicines that would offer temporary relief without ever addressing the source. For my parents and their contemporaries, their pills were just a Band-Aid disguising but never really getting to the real cause of their ill health and discomfort. Actually, in those days, my parents were not considered to be unhealthy. They were just like everyone else who had high blood pressure, high cholesterol, and fatigue. These were supposedly the normal and therefore acceptable results of aging, or so they thought.

When Cynthia came to see me last August, it was by default. She had recently been to see her internist for an annual checkup, and he was concerned by her apparent increase in blood pressure and her LDL cholesterol. His concern mounted to alarm when he realized that Cynthia had just celebrated her thirtieth birthday—hardly someone who should be dealing with the ominous markers for challenged health.

When we met in my office for her initial visit, Cynthia seemed more interested in the fifteen pounds she had put on than these other symptoms. She complained that the overweight was historical: She had been putting it on and taking it off for the past ten years. But this time around, she'd been unable to lose it, not even using her sister's diet tactics: a week of eating grapefruit, drinking lots of diet soda, and going over the top by spending every day working out at the gym. All to no avail. The weight wouldn't budge from around her middle. When I asked her if she had mentioned this weight issue to her physician she'd said no, why would she talk about her weight with her doctor? She was already doing what he had suggested, eating less and exercising more.

Thankfully for Cynthia, her internist did make the connection between her increase in blood pressure and cholesterol levels and her diet and nutrition habits, and so she wound up in the chair opposite me. I was glad the doctor suggested this visit because such conditions can be too quickly treated with drugs. In Cynthia's case, as in many cases of high blood pressure and cholesterol, changes in diet and nutrition are enough to reverse the high levels, even for those stubborn genetic apple-doesn't-fall-far-from-the-tree types.

As I listened to Cynthia, I felt that we were once again dealing with the same telltale symptoms. At thirty years old, Cynthia said she had been battling her weight her whole life, watching her waist balloon and deflate right in front of her eyes. But her most compelling complaint was that she constantly felt exhausted—emotionally as well as physically—and now she possessed the clear markers of aging at a relatively young age, markers that can

> Ponce de Leon was looking for the Fountain of Youth. Proper insulin function may just lead us to it.

be delayed well into the seventies or eighties, if not forever. Aging does not have to be synonymous with disease.

If Cynthia's story seems at all familiar, then let's go to the heart of the problem: eliminating your insulin resistance and reteaching your body to let insulin into the cells.

DO SOMETHING BEFORE IT'S TOO LATE

Historically, treatment for this crafty cluster of conditions (the high blood pressure, high cholesterol, high blood sugar, high triglycerides) has been based on dietary recommendations and medications. For too long, everyone in the medical community focused aggressive treatment for patients with heart trouble only *after* their clients had already suffered from a heart attack. The same approach was used toward people with type 2 diabetes; never mind that many of their patients had been exhibiting symptoms for years before they developed the actual disease. Happily, our modern medical community has begun to recognize the link between the factors of the Metabolic Mix-Up and these illnesses. Many health practitioners have done a 180 and now support strong treatment for the at-risk client *before* it's too late.

This news was such a change from protocol that it made the cover story of *The New York Times* on May 16, 2001. According to the article, a national panel sponsored by the U.S. government announced that heart disease and heart attacks, the two leading killers in the United States, could be reduced significantly by people changing their diets and by ingesting cholesterol-lowering pills.

Now we know pills are not enough; with our new understanding, we have advanced our thinking and realize that we can actually orchestrate our bodies to do what they were designed to do: allow the glucose cargo into the cells. Aiding and abetting the metabolism of our food is how we talk to our chemistry. The Carb-Careful Solution shows you how.

Following this program, you will eat in a new and different way, reducing the amount of carbohydrates in your diet, introducing them as late in the day as possible (preferably at dinner), and making sure you're eating carbs in the company of quality proteins and vegetables. In this way, your body begins to release insulin in a more balanced, regulated way. Note that I say *reduce* carbohydrates, not replace altogether. This approach works when you eat from all of the food groups: protein, complex carbs, veggies, and yes, even fat. And make sure to drink plenty of water. Water not only mobilizes fat but it is also critical in the proper metabolism of all the foods you eat.

This reasonable and more moderate approach to diet and nutrition has now become mainstream. In another Sunday *New York Times Magazine* cover story on July 7, 2002, entitled "What if Fat Doesn't Make Us Fat?," the author presents the most recent research on the dangers of carbohydrates, linking the overreliance on carbs to the growing obesity and diabetes epidemic as well as to insulin resistance, the main cause of both problems. Carbs can make you sick!

You are also going to learn how supplements have the ability to change the nature of your cells, an incredible opportunity when you really think about it. Supplements of vitamins, minerals, and other compounds also help increase insulin sensitivity and allow you to process carbohydrates that normally would trigger your Metabolic Mix-Up.

Finally, you will see how exercise is a miracle touch that can increase the fire under your heels. I always find that when people understand why they should do something and it makes sense, they are more likely to accept the suggestion and try to make the change. Amazingly, it doesn't take much exercise to reap the benefits. You can start by walking for fifteen minutes three times a week. Just get moving. This is enough to begin to help sensitize your cells so that they allow more of the insulin cargo in. It's like a bicycle whose chain needs to be oiled; one minute it's in the garage gathering dust and rust, and the next minute, after a little oil and TLC, you're out biking like you were a kid again.

That's what exercise is like for your body's cells—a reprogramming to perform in a fantastic new way.

And together supplements and exercise will begin to improve your body composition, which is absolutely vital to good health. I'm not talking about weight (or losing weight); I'm talking about achieving the best lean body mass to body fat ratio as possible. Supplements and exercise help you reshape your body so that you continue your quest for vital health and increased longevity.

By combining each of these ingredients—balancing your blood sugar, controlling your carb intake, supplements, and exercise—you've got a powerful, multifaceted device to isolate and eradicate your insulin-resistant chemistry, creating the momentum to abolish your Metabolic Mix-Up forever! All you need to do is begin the four steps and you will soon feel more alive and present in your life than you ever thought possible.

CHAPTER 3

Do You Have the Metabolic Mix-Up?

IT'S UP TO YOU

It's an old adage, but it's true; if you've got your health, you've got everything . . . so guard it. Protect it. Nurture it. You wash your car once a week, you take a shower every morning, you're careful to watch your bank account when outside forces affect it. Why don't more of us pay this kind of attention to the ways our bodies feel, change, and react?

Spending time to secure quality health is the most important investment you'll ever make, and yet powerful forces can often keep us away from taking a firm hold of this responsibility. If insulin resistance was knocking on your door, wouldn't you want to know about it? Who says we can't predict the future? It's really in your hands. You have the power to change the course of your chemistry, and your physical, emotional, and mental destiny.

Before we go any further in our quest for vibrant health, let's find out if you have or are at risk of developing the Metabolic Mix-Up. As you know by now, this powerful metabolic disturbance has quite ordinary-seeming characteristics that may not be getting your attention. Do these sound like you?

> ## CHECK WITH YOUR DOCTOR
>
> Never go off your medications without your doctor's approval. By taming your Metabolic Mix-Up with the Carb-Careful Solution, you should eventually curb your need for medications. Do not stop or change the dose of any medication without your doctor's approval.

THE FOUR RISK FACTORS

There are four areas of your life that contribute to your chemical betrayal. Let's explore this territory and see how we can open the door to your Metabolic Mix-Up in order to tame it once and for all.

1. your family history
2. your physical condition—weight, blood pressure, cholesterol
3. your eating habits—diet
4. your lifestyle—exercise

By evaluating these four areas of your life, you can not only assess to what degree you have the Metabolic Mix-Up but you can also determine what factors are contributing the most to how you feel. Remember, even a child can develop this disorder of metabolism and run the risk of life-threatening diseases, as evidenced by the younger and younger members of the type 2 diabetes category. Wouldn't you want to know if you are at risk? Better yet, don't you want to know an effective, valuable solution to tame the tiresome triggers once and for all so that you don't unwittingly take the risk of developing the major diseases that were once only associated with aging?

Your Family History: Evaluating Your Inheritance

Why was I a Sugar Baby? Not simply because I loved to stop for a chocolate-filled doughnut on the way home from school on Fridays, but because I was brought up in a box of cookies and my parents lived in and decorated that box of cookies. You know how we hope our new baby will have Uncle Ray's blue eyes or Aunt Helen's fair skin? It's all in that box of cookies. We all know the power of genes to predetermine eye color, hairline, height, and nose shape. But did you know you can also be genetically predisposed to crave sugar and starch? And right after this inherited craving comes an inherited glitch in your ability to metabolize the sweets and starches you crave.

It would be nearly impossible to do a genetic screening of yourself, but you can do a review of your family's medical history. This information will help you begin to gather clues as to what conditions run in your family and how these conditions may have been inherited by you.

Let's look at your family tree to see which branch may be yours:

1. Do you rationalize your higher-than-you-would-like cholesterol as a family trait like the regal height you inherited from Uncle Henry and Grandma Mae?
2. Is type 2 diabetes a close cousin in your family?
3. Has anyone in your family died of heart disease or a heart attack?
4. Does either of your parents suffer from high blood pressure?
5. Does either of your parents share your tendency to put weight around the middle?
6. Has your brother or sister had to take cholesterol-lowering medication even after following a low-fat-almost-vegetarian diet?
7. When you were growing up, was the most important question, "What's for dinner?" followed quickly by, "What's for dessert?"

8. Do you and your family members share high triglyceride levels as if they were golf handicaps?

Use this information to find out whether your increasing blood pressure and LDL levels may be related to *your* Metabolic Mix-Up. If you come up with a lot of people in your family sharing these traits, chances are that your high blood pressure has more to do with insulin resistance than high salt intake. So instead of being treated individually with high cholesterol or high blood pressure medications, it is more important that you begin to deal directly with the root cause—your insulin resistance.

We live in a culture where it has been traditional to treat problems individually—one pill for your high blood pressure and another one for your high cholesterol and yet another one for your anxiety. Each of the body's systems may be programmed to carry out its own specific task, but they all work synergistically with one another to create a whole that is greater than all its individual parts. The fact that you have high cholesterol and high blood pressure, are often fatigued, and crave carbohydrates is not a coincidence. It's a direct result of your compromised metabolism.

For those of you who have not yet expressed the genes of your family tree, take this as the midnight warning of Paul Revere: Something is afoot. Your health is in danger. Talk to your health-care practitioner and ask him or her to review your history with your Metabolic Mix-Up in mind so that you can develop an accurate perspective on the status of your physical condition.

Your Body, Your Self: Evaluating Your Physical Condition

How do you really feel? Is your body in tip-top shape? Can you walk a mile with ease? Can you climb a flight of stairs without feeling winded? Do you accept feeling just okay rather than great?

Below is a list of questions that may be beginning to seem familiar. As you become more and more aware of the characteristics of the Metabolic Mix-Up, you're even closer to determining whether you are one of the 16 to 20 million people of the walking wounded, living a life that is less than vibrant, not knowing if you already may be on your way to type 2 diabetes.

1. Does the sugar call-of-the-wild make you consider trading your beloved baseball ticket for your favorite dessert?
2. Do you have high cholesterol?
3. Has your blood pressure sharply increased recently?
4. Do you have an apple figure that looks and feels like you wear a tire around your middle?
5. Do you have strong smelling or deep yellow-colored urine?
6. Has your glucose level been getting higher marks in your blood tests?
7. If you are a woman, do you often experience menstrual difficulties?
8. Are you often fatigued and irritable throughout the day?
9. Are you often wakeful in the middle of the night?
10. If you are a woman, do you tend to have acne and hair in unwanted places, signaling polycystic ovaries?
11. Do all your old favorite dieting tricks for controlling those upsetting five to ten extra pounds no longer work?

What a catch-22: You feel tired all day but can't sleep at night. If this sounds like you—even a few nights a week or month—then something is up with your diet and nutrition. If you are consistently irritable and tired, these are reliable signs that your chemistry is out of whack and you need to balance your blood

---

TAKE TWO STRAWBERRIES AND CALL ME IN THE MORNING!

If you find yourself tossing and turning, tired but too restless to sleep, you made need a blood sugar boost. Try eating two strawberries to balance your blood sugar and take away that restless feeling, enabling you to sleep.

ASK YOUR DOCTOR

These are the tests you should talk to your physician about:

- homocysteine levels
- triglycerides
- HDL and LDL cholesterol
- blood pressure
- glucose tolerance with corresponding insulin levels
- ferritin levels (iron)
- uric acid levels

sugar and replenish your body with other vital nutrients. Clearly your body is telling you it needs more energy. And don't think that diet soda or extra cup of coffee is going to do the trick. In an hour or so, you'll be back to feeling low and miserable, wishing you could take a long siesta. But you probably also know that in spite of your fatigue, that your low blood sugar that you set up earlier in the day will cause you to have even more restless sleep. The brain, desperate for its glucose, will make you feel restless and wakeful.

Paying close attention to how you feel, check to see if you have the two most common physiological indicators of the Metabolic Mix-Up: high blood pressure and high cholesterol (specifically a high LDL level). Even if you are only in your thirties you should have these levels checked by your health practitioner. Blood pressure measures how hard your heart has to work to pump blood into the arteries and through your circulatory system. A blood pressure of 140/90 or lower is considered normal, while 120/80 is the ideal. The higher (systolic) number represents the pressure when the heart is beating while the lower (diastolic) number represents the pressure when the heart is resting between beats. High blood pressure, also called hypertension, places you at risk for heart attack and stroke. When it exists with obesity and smoking, high blood cholesterol levels can sky-rocket.

**ASK YOUR DOCTOR ABOUT YOUR
HOMOCYSTEINE LEVELS**

Homocysteine is a particular amino acid that can build up in your blood. Excessive amounts are now considered to be as much an indication for heart disease as cholesterol levels.

High levels of cholesterol in the blood increase the amount of plaque in the arteries and can lead to heart disease. A total blood cholesterol level under 200 mg/dL is desirable, lowering your risk for heart disease and diabetes. Whether your cholesterol is high or not, your physician will most likely test the individual levels of LDL (bad cholesterol) and HDL (good cholesterol)—the ideal target for LDL is lower than 110 mg/dL and for HDL is greater than 50 mg/dL. A high level of LDL increases your risk of heart disease as does a low level of HDL, which has protective benefits for the heart.

The Apple Doesn't Fall Far from the Tree: Evaluating Your Weight and Shape

All of us gain weight in our special way. But those of us who tend to put on weight in exactly the same place—around our middle—are blessed (cursed is more like it) with an apple figure. Do you eat two cookies or a bag of popcorn and it suddenly appears like a loaf of bread around your middle? You're one of us! Years ago it would have been devastating to belong to this group because membership would have meant inevitable craving and a future destined to pudginess—lifelong chemical insurrection and

THE UNRELENTING INSULIN INSULT

Insulin resistance accelerates the progression of atherosclerosis, a process whereby layers of yellowish plaque made up of cholesterol, fats, and other particles build up in the walls of arteries. As the arteries narrow, blood flow slows and the blood vessels may become blocked. This can lead to coronary artery disease, heart attack, or stroke.

The other factors to look for in a general diagnostic review are high uric acid in your urine, which is usually looked at as an indicator of gout, and high ferritin (iron), and, for women, polycystic ovaries. But in the case of tracking down the clues for your Metabolic Mix-Up, high uric acid can indicate insulin resistance. Another important factor is fasting blood sugar ratio of less than 4.5.

Women who experience irregular menstrual cycles (heavy or irregular bleeding) should also be wary. While these situations may not be directly linked to a Metabolic Mix-Up, it's best to check out any possible relationship. I'd rather you be safe rather than sorry.

You may find that one or two or even three of these factors are part of your profile, and just another indication that you need to read further to see if you have more conditions that can help you identify the full extent of your Metabolic Mix-Up. You have the power to learn how to strengthen, reverse, and better your physical condition in order to eliminate these side effects of your metabolic disorder.

a round body that are the result of your attachment to all those sweet little starchy devils.

Now don't get lost in bad feelings about yourself or in fears that you can't break the cycle. Just be aware. This tendency to carry your formerly trim waist in layers of fat is a sure sign that you are *very* reactive to carbohydrates and have difficulty processing these foods. If these foods aren't metabolized properly, then your body can't use them for fuel; and if your body doesn't use them, then it stores them as fat. Right around your middle!

One client of mine told me of an upcoming costume party. Patting her tummy, she exclaimed, "The only costume I can wear to the masquerade party is to go as the Pillsbury Doughboy and everyone will know it's me. No matter what I do, I can't seem to lose it!" Do you sometimes awaken so puffy even though you fit into your small jeans just three days before? Can your belt buckle travel two holes in the wrong direction the morning after a carb fest? If so, you need to watch the tendency to put weight around your middle as a warning.

This apple-shaped figure means you have a high waist-to-hip ratio, another definitive indicator of the Metabolic Mix-Up. The ratio is calculated by dividing your waist size by hip size. If you have a 30-inch waistline and hip measurements of 40 inches, your ratio would be 0.75. Women with a ratio above 0.8 more than likely have the Metabolic Mix-Up.

BEER BELLIES BEWARE!

Evidence reports that beer belly types are more at risk for heart disease. This kind of extra weight is the calling card of the Metabolic Mix-Up. This apple-shaped figure is usually an indication of too much body fat with too little muscle.

THE BEAUTY OF THE BMI

There is another way to determine if your weight is getting in your way: the BMI. Your body mass index (BMI) determines if your weight is healthy for your height and general physique. BMI is calculated by dividing your weight in kilograms (1 kilogram equals 2.2 pounds) by your height in meters squared (1 meter equals 39.37 inches). But don't worry about complicated mathematical formulas; you can determine your BMI by using the chart below.

A BMI of 18.5 to 24.9 is considered normal while a measurement of 25 to 29.9 is overweight and 30 or higher is obese. Heart disease, diabetes, stroke, arthritis, and some cancers are just a few of the serious health risks associated with a high BMI.

Being overweight is only part of the problem. It is the distribution of weight (the apple figure as measured by the BMI) that is the real calling card of the Metabolic Mix-Up, as well as an *inability* to lose weight. It's fair to say that many women and men come to see me because they want to lose weight. And while I want to and can help them achieve this, I try to get them to develop a wider, more inclusive focus. Being overweight is often a symptom; it's not the root of the problem. And when clients shift their focus from losing weight to getting healthy and eating right, they not only lose the weight more easily, they also learn to eat in a way that is life saving for their bodies. Yes, you will be able to keep off those unwanted pounds forever, but more than that, you will discover a way to live to your fullest potential.

Determining Your Body Mass Index (BMI)

The table opposite has already done the math and metric conversions. To use the table, find the appropriate height in the left-hand column. Move across the row to the given weight. The number at the top of the column is the BMI for that height and weight.

Do You Have the Metabolic Mix-Up?

BMI (kg/m²)	19	20	21	22	23	24	25	26	27	28	29	30	35	40
Height (in.)							Weight (lb.)							
58	91	96	100	105	110	115	119	124	129	134	138	143	167	191
59	94	99	104	109	114	119	124	128	133	138	143	148	173	198
60	97	102	107	112	118	123	128	133	138	143	148	153	179	204
61	100	106	111	116	122	127	132	137	143	148	153	158	185	211
62	104	109	115	120	126	131	136	142	147	153	158	164	191	218
63	107	113	118	124	130	135	141	146	152	158	163	169	197	225
64	110	116	122	128	134	140	145	151	157	163	169	174	204	232
65	114	120	126	132	138	144	150	156	162	168	174	180	210	240
66	118	124	130	136	142	148	155	161	167	173	179	186	216	247
67	121	127	134	140	146	153	159	166	172	178	185	191	223	255
68	125	131	138	144	151	158	164	171	177	184	190	197	230	262
69	128	135	142	149	155	162	169	176	182	189	196	203	236	270
70	132	139	146	153	160	167	174	181	188	195	202	207	243	278
71	136	143	150	157	165	172	179	186	193	200	208	215	250	286
72	140	147	154	162	169	177	184	191	199	206	213	221	258	294
73	144	151	159	166	174	182	189	197	204	212	219	227	265	302
74	148	155	163	171	179	186	194	202	210	218	225	233	272	311
75	152	160	168	176	184	192	200	208	216	224	232	240	279	319
76	156	164	172	180	189	197	205	213	221	230	238	246	287	328

POWER PROFILE

As you become more familiar with your personal profile, you need to keep track of your various measurements and blood levels. Here are the targets to aspire to:

Target blood pressure: 120/80
Target HDL cholesterol: greater than 50 mg
Target LDL cholesterol: lower than 110 mg
Target triglycerides: fewer than 150 mg/dL
Target ferritin level: 30/380
Target glucose level: 70 to 110 mg/dL
Target body mass index: 18.5 to 24.9
Target waist-to-hip ratio: 0.8 or lower

WHAT ARE YOU *REALLY* EATING? EVALUATING YOUR EATING HABITS

You can change your life, but first you must be willing to examine your lifestyle. Are you really paying attention to what you eat? Do you decide on Monday that you will eat healthier—less fat and more fruit and vegetables—only to find yourself on an all-fruit diet on Thursday in a desperate attempt to look good at the Friday night party? Do you have erratic eating patterns—bingeing one day and dieting the next on "healthy" carbohydrate foods? Or are you eating sushi, knowing that your restaurant has safe fish but ignoring the fact that it's wrapped around a starchy white rice bundle?

Answer these true or false:

1. You always find yourself jumping into bread, cake, cereal, cookies, or pasta.
2. One roll, one cracker, one of anything is seldom enough; you usually want lots more.

3. You could describe yourself as a yo-yo dieter.
4. French fries and ketchup are more important than the hamburger.
5. You barely finish your bag of popcorn before extra layers are nesting around your middle.
6. After a carbohydrate overload, you gain weight with frightening speed.
7. You lost weight last month but you're at a plateau.
8. You can't eat cereal without a banana.
9. You never say no to a bagel.
10. Desserts on the menu catch your eye before entrees.
11. Every meal must have a starch to feel complete.
12. If there's bread on the table, it doesn't stay there very long.
13. A hamburger without a bun is like a man without a country.
14. Every day deserves an afternoon candy bar.
15. Once you drink a glass of wine, you want more—of everything!

How many trues does it take to give you the blueprint for the mix-up? If you answered an enthusiastic true to several questions, you may be an active participant in triggering the cravings that keep your Metabolic Mix-Up going. Remember how a blood sugar imbalance (the end result of the Metabolic Mix-Up) causes an uncontrollable, endless desire for carbohydrates? These cravings can be stopped, but first you have to control your blood sugar.

Did you ever realize how powerful food can be? As if the chemical calling were not bad enough, we have learned to use food like a drug when feelings flood in. Does depression feel like a bag of cookies is in order, without even questioning whether you're genuinely hungry or not? You have lots of company. You're not alone. So many people have learned to use food to block their feelings, replacing sorrow or other strong, often sad, emotions with the familiar, delicious distraction of food. It sure beats feeling those upsetting feelings. But like the mesmerizing bottles in my parents' medicine chest that only addressed the surface of these problems, not the root, food will not replace a broken heart or a broken carburetor.

You should be getting the picture by now: It's easy to trigger to the mix-up when you have the genetic predisposition in addition to poor eating habits. So unless you want to be controlled by your chemistry for the rest of your life, you need to take steps right now to redesign your eating habits and adopt a new approach to food.

STOP THE EQUATION FOR DISASTER

The Metabolic Mix-Up can be caused by either a genetic predisposition or poor eating habits—or both. But if you follow the Carb-Careful Solution, you will quiet your genes and say goodbye to trigger-craving empty meals!

HOW ACTIVE ARE YOU? EVALUATING EXERCISE IN YOUR LIFE

I have not forgotten about exercise; I've just been waiting to ask: How much are you actually getting? Many clients hope that I will ignore this last factor altogether, thinking that lowering their fat and calorie intake will do it all. And, with the Metabolic Mix-Up wreaking havoc on their bodies, they do not have any energy to spare.

Please take this warning to heart: A person at risk for insulin resistance cannot succeed without getting off that couch even if he or she reduces the number of calories he or she eats. The key to greater freedom is to include exercise in your life. You can eat more, enjoy more, experience greater ease and peace of mind while continuing to lose weight if you begin to exercise regularly.

The impact of exercise on insulin receptors is dramatic and known. Type 1 diabetics know that they require less insulin if they exercise regularly because the exercise helps their bodies utilize the insulin more effectively. Exercise has an analogous effect on those of us with the Metabolic Mix-Up. The more frequently we exercise, the more receptive our cells become to insulin. That's right! You can actually recondition your cells to behave properly. Exercise is a powerful tool in our fight to vanquish the insulin insult by changing your body at a cellular level.

With a more active lifestyle, you don't have to express those genes that will interfere with a less than vibrant life. Exercise will let you wear your thin jeans as though you had thin genes not just because you are burning calories but because you are redirecting your chemistry, enhancing your metabolism, and improving your body composition.

And fear not! I don't mean you have to get up and run a mile every morning before work. You can start slowly. And make it fun—exercise doesn't have to be a chore or a labor. I don't want you to stress about how to exercise or how to fit it into your already busy schedule. In Chapter eight, you will learn many of the techniques my clients have used so well, making exercise an enjoyable part of your life.

THE EXERCISE EQUATION

When you exercise just twenty minutes a day, four times per week, you give your heart a boost. The more you exercise, the more you condition your cells' receptivity to insulin, slowly but surely reversing your insulin resistance.

THE MIND-BODY CONNECTION

We all know that when we feel bad physically, we also can feel it emotionally. Just the other day, Steven, a very successful banker, came into my office completely frustrated and depressed. He'd just spent the weekend dodging sweets and starches at a couple of parties only to return home on Sunday night and go through a pint of ice cream—and that was after three slices of pizza. Not only had he triggered his insulin-resistant body but he also reinforced the insult even further by craving more carbohydrates and making himself feel even more lethargic. And, as if *that* were not enough, his emotional well-being plummeted with his blood sugar. Instead of giving himself comfort, he was giving himself more reasons to be depressed.

This tender connection between how we feel in our bodies and in our minds is why the Carb-Careful Solution is geared just as much to your mental well-being as to your physical well-being. One client, Suzanne, had been in a deep depression for years. She was grossly overweight and had tried every fad diet on the market but to no avail. Within four weeks on the program, she lost ten pounds and dropped her cholesterol fifty-three points. This new Suzanne, who had described her exercise program as walking to and from her car, was now walking half an hour a day. She fit it in at lunch time at the mall or any place she could. But the aspect of the program that she was happiest about was not the weight she shed but how she felt. "For the first time in ten years, I look forward to getting out of bed in the morning. I'm interested in life again. I know I still have a ways to go to getting to my ideal weight, but now I'm going to enjoy the journey."

BLUE GENES

Blue genes may well be the results of your Metabolic Mix-Up, indicating that you may have inherited the tendency to feel blue or moody. But you don't have to express your genes: Good food, good life, supplements, and exercise all can help you control the expression of your genetic wiring, ensuring your potential for joy in living.

Suzanne took back her life by taking control of her health, and you can too! This is the ultimate act of self-love. Unfortunately, the word *diet* has become linked with the idea of doing without, and taking care of yourself has meant deprivation and misery. It's time to take care of your future. Settle down and stop looking for silver bullets. You need to take charge of how you eat, move, and think so that you discover the vibrant life you deserve. It's time to stop flitting from one program to another and commit to the formula that will work for you: the Carb–Careful Solution.

Think about the program as a gift, a way to truly take care of yourself and enhance your life. Once you learn what to eat and when, you will begin to control your chemistry and feel life humming through you.

By strengthening your body in this way, you will turn back your body's clock, reducing your biological age and increasing your health.

Welcome to your future!

Walking the Steps

—∞∞∞—

Get Ready for Your Great Adventure

THE SYNERGY OF THE FOUR STEPS

The program's four steps give you the tools to balance your blood sugar, further control your carbohydrate intake, include important vitamin and mineral supplements every day, and add exercise to your regular routine, all of which are crucial to reversing your insulin resistance and minimizing your Metabolic Mix-Up.

Remember, you can't be a bystander in this program. The Carb-Careful Solution is a dynamic approach to eating and health: I'm giving you the information, and it's up to you to monitor your responses, watching for both positive and negative changes in your energy level and other specific side effects. It will not be hard to recognize an increase in vitality or a drop in energy level.

Here are the four steps and their specific goals. Once you get started, you will be building momentum with each day, with each step.

STEP ONE: BASIC BALANCE
- Achieve blood sugar control
- Diminish your carbohydrate cravings
- Flush the body of toxins and hydrate the body

STEP TWO: CARB-CAREFUL
- Reduce carbohydrates at specific times to stop the insulin damage
- Control glucose release from carbohydrates
- Lock in better balance

STEP THREE: SUPPLEMENT SOLUTION
Introduce vitamin, mineral, and herbal supplements to:
- Burn fat
- Support immune system
- Enable you to reintroduce some carbohydrates into your diet
- Improve cell's acceptance of insulin

STEP FOUR: EXERCISE EUPHORIA
- Begin personal exercise regime
- Reverse insulin resistance at cellular level
- Lose weight if desired
- Aid metabolism of carbs

When the sum total is greater than the parts, you create synergy and that's exactly what happens when you walk the four steps. It's the parts as a whole (the four steps themselves) that help you to escort the insulin into the cells—whether you're first doing Basic Balance, recovering from a rebound, or accepting the challenge of Carb-Careful. Like a thousand-piece jigsaw puzzle, if you're missing a few pieces, the whole won't hang together. But when you pop in those vital four pieces, you can pick up the puzzle, frame it, show it, and walk it around the room. That's the power of synergy. These steps build on one another, working together to create a force that will take you from living life at half-mast to living life with joie de vivre. No longer held back by your compromised chemistry, your body will now be able to function at a higher level, and you will feel the result of vibrant health.

As Matthew said, "It's so easy. If you had told me when I walked in that I would do this without a thought, I wouldn't have believed you! It has just become a part of me—I guess that's what you mean by owning the diet!" 'Are you ready for your great adventure?

IT'S YOUR GREAT ADVENTURE

Okay—so now you're ready to take some concrete steps to great health and creating a happier you. Don't be nervous. I know it's going to work; it already has for thousands of women and men just like you. And the reason why is simple: The Carb-Careful Solution is doable and livable. These four steps will make you feel so much better—physically, mentally, and emotionally—that you will need no convincing from me to stick with it. With the very first step, you will begin to experience the impact of the changes you are making, and these changes will soon become an easy part of your life. Please don't hesitate to try because you are going to respond to what you are doing and love the results. And if you don't feel dramatically better, well then you just won't do it. But experience is the best teacher, so I know you will want this program to be a part of your new, vibrant life.

One of my clients, Barbara, came to see me so depleted of energy that she was certain she had the beginning of some disease. "I've been tired before, but I know this is not normal. I feel so lifeless that I have two states of being—I'm either sleeping or I'm irritable. Together we discussed her recent climb in blood pressure and LDL cholesterol, as well as some overweight she wanted to shed. We went over the first two steps of the program—Basic Balance and Carb-Careful—and within just a few weeks, she appeared in my office a new person! "I used to spend half my day preparing for an evening out, trying to save my energy so that I could enjoy a movie," she explained. "Now I just live my life, and when I want to go to the movies, I just go! I don't have to overthink it anymore." She became even more excited when she heard that this dramatic shift in her energy was directly related to changing her foods. "This is the best thing I've ever done. Even though it still seems strange that my blood pressure is going down because I gave up my bread. It used to be my favorite food, but now I have no craving for it whatsoever. I also don't have any interest in my old favorites that I used to binge on. I am elevated—it's unbelievable. As a matter of fact, people are asking me what I am doing. My clothing is much looser. I seem to be shrinking in a good way. I talk to *everyone* about this program."

Did I mention that Barbara is in her seventies?

For Barbara, the first step to regaining her energy was to stop her cravings and get her blood sugar under control. Once she was able to calm her insulin activity, Barbara was on her way. And I know that Barbara will continue to look and feel this well as long as she continues to walk the steps and pays attention to this new way of approaching food. The program is an insurance policy to keep her blood work numbers in control—a concrete tool to ensure a youthful future.

This program is not just about learning to give yourself nutrients or good calories; it is more about the third dimension of chemistry. What will the juice you drink at breakfast invite you to do in the afternoon? It's about beginning to redirect your chemistry. Once you balance your blood sugar and lock it into place, you won't crave or fall into mood swings that leave you feeling lethargic and exhausted.

In the beginning, you may think about your foods a lot. After all, you will be trading one style of eating for another, so be patient. After a few weeks, you won't have to think so much about the foods. It will become the way you do things, as natural as showering in the morning, taking your dog for a walk, or hugging your child. At first, you may find yourself pouring over your Giant Food List in the next chapter and worrying about walking the steps. Please don't worry. The next four chapters lay out the program step-by-step so you don't have to memorize anything. All you need to do is read ahead. I promise this new way of eating will make sense soon. I can't tell you how many clients have said this to me over the years. And when I hear, "It just makes sense, Adele," I know something has clicked inside.

That man or woman is ready to travel the road to real health. And for Barbara—bless her heart—she is helping to spread the word. Younger or older, it's never too late to try something new.

THE BASICS OF WALKING THE STEPS

I know I am asking you to do things differently. But if you keep doing the same old things you will keep the same old problems. Once you feel the changes in your body, your mind, bolstered by that new-found energy, will lead you to a new joy for living. You will look back at your old self and see how uplifted you've become and how incredibly, naturally comfortable you feel within yourself. This is my promise to you. All you have to do is follow the steps.

Before we get into the details of each step, you will learn the components of the Carb-Careful Solution.

• **Put together the best plate.** This tool will help you focus on how to combine your foods so that you get the most nutrients with the least risk of triggering your insulin resistance.

• **Use your Giant Food List.** This enormous list of foods (at the end of this chapter) ranks and organizes foods so that you know how to choose the best foods and how to avoid the foods that may trigger your Metabolic Mix-Up.

• **Eat a reasonable range of portion sizes and amounts.** You will learn how to determine a reasonable amount of food for yourself by checking the reasonable range diagrams on page 63–64. You will be freed from time-consuming weighing and measuring.

• **Time your meals and snacks.** You will learn that you must eat regularly throughout the day in order to keep your chemistry in check—preferably in two- to three-hour intervals. If you don't eat three meals a day and at least two snacks at regular intervals, then you risk triggering the mix-up.

• **Tap into the miracle of water.** Did you know that water makes up more than half of your total body weight? You need plenty of water just to keep your body functioning. Water not only mobilizes fat to help in weight loss but it also helps to deliver valuable nutrients throughout the body. It is of critical importance that you drink plenty of water while on the program—ten glasses a day is a minimum requirement. But try for twelve!

• **Keep a journal.** Your journal will become your best friend, helping you stay aware, a place where you can realistically keep track of your experiences as you walk the steps.

PUTTING TOGETHER THE BEST PLATE

The golden rule for those of us with the Metabolic Mix-Up is simple but powerful: The food you eat plays an enormous role in how you feel. This golden rule forms the backbone of the program. It informs what you eat, how you eat, at which times you eat, and even how you think about eating. I cannot emphasize enough that *all* food groups are essential. It's when you eat a combination of *high-quality proteins, nonstarchy (complex) carbs,* lots of *veggies,* which are complex carbohydrates, *minimal saturated fats,* and lots of *fiber,* that you lessen your chances for triggering your mix-up and pave the way for vibrant health. These nutrient sources are built into the diet and incorporated into the Giant Food List (see pages 93–103), so you don't have to worry about memorizing this information. But it is important that you know how I've assembled the Giant Food List so that when you put together your plate, you select the best foods and create the most interesting menus.

COMPLEX CARBOHYDRATES
Carbohydrates fuel the brain. Although your brain represents less than 3 percent of your total body weight, it consumes nearly 20 percent of the blood sugar in your body, and carbs are your main source of blood sugar. When you choose complex carbs, which are nutrient laden, instead of simple carbs or sugars, you fuel your brain without triggering your Metabolic Mix-Up.

VEGGIES

Veggies are carbohydrates; yet they are high in fiber and low in glucose so they are absorbed more slowly than starchy carbs. This way the brain and body get their nutrients without awakening your insulin-resistant chemistry. Veggies are also rich in other nutrients such as betacarotene, vitamin C, and flavones.

FIBER

Fiber slows down the absorption of carbohydrates, helping reduce the call for insulin. The more fiber in the carbohydrate, the more powerfully you control your chemistry.

HIGH-QUALITY PROTEIN

Your body needs protein for cell growth, revitalization of your nervous system and muscles, and as a regulating agent in the breakdown and placement of carbs. The more careful you are to choose foods that have the highest degree of protein with the least amount of saturated or bad fat, the more power you give your body.

ESSENTIAL FATTY ACIDS (EFAs)

EFAs are essential to controlling your chemistry. Essential fatty acids are not the rich, thick fats you'll find attached to deep-fried chicken or embedded in chocolate frosting. These are the fats that you *need*—omega-3 and omega-6 oils to keep your skin glowing, your hair shiny, and more important, to reduce blood pressure, triglyceride levels, and blood clot formations.

CARB-CAREFUL FOOD FACTS

Here are some basics you need to know:

• **You need carbs—but you need to understand them, too.** You don't have to eat a carb-*free* diet. There are many pure-power and middle-road carbs that deliver valuable nutrients. You just have to be smart and use your reasonable range guide and eat foods in proper combination.

• **Simple sugars and complex carbohydrates are the two main types of carbohydrates we eat in our diet.** Although similar, these two types differ in complexity and size. Complex carbohydrates are more slowly digested and assimilated by the body than simple carbohydrates, or sugars. Try to become familiar with these types because they differ in their rate of absorption, which plays an important role in the way insulin responds to a meal. The more complex, the less they will impact your system, helping you avoid the boomerang effect of blood sugar imbalance.

The simple sugars, on the other hand, should carry a warning label: Since they are more rapidly absorbed, they create an emergency call for excessive insulin. Strangely enough, the result can either be a low blood sugar effect after eating, which is called hypoglycemia, or too much blood sugar, which is called hyperglycemia. Don't be fooled into thinking that all complex carbs are your friends. They also come in two different forms—refined or unrefined. Refined, such as those found in processed food, act like simple sugars. The more unrefined a complex carbohydrate, the more fiber it has and the better it is for your metabolic health.

Vegetables are perfect examples of unrefined complex carbohydrates—high in fiber and rich in nutritious value. And the ever-present white bread is a star example of a simple sugar. Even well-meaning, nutritionally wise parents can wind up giving in to their child's attachment to white flour, making the strongest adult a minor at mealtime when faced with a toddler's closed mouth. This is why I like to switch the old order and introduce vegetables before fruit to an infant's innocent palate. Do you know *anyone* who will eat their string beans once they've had some warm apple pie?

• **You need to eat foods that eat insulin.** Foods that specifically improve the body's ability to use insulin include deepwater fish, such as salmon, sardines, and mackerel; flaxseed; and omega-3 oils. Try grinding up flaxseeds in a mini-grinder for best results. But if you're not eating any of these foods two or three times a week, then be sure to take your supplements.

• **You need to eat good fats and restrict saturated fats.** The good fats (essential fatty acids) are necessary for normal reproduction and growth. They are converted into prostaglandins (a hormone), which regulate all body functions at the cellular level. Prostaglandins control blood pressure, clotting, inflammation, allergies, sodium, water excretion, and tumor growth, among other functions. However, foods high in saturated fat should be eaten very sparingly since they can interfere with your body's ability to use insulin.

• **Whole foods are wholesome.** The more unprocessed (i.e., *whole*) a food is, the more fiber it contains and the harder it is for your body to break it down. The harder to break down, the more slowly the insulin is released; and the more slowly insulin is released, the more chance your body has to metabolize food properly and regulate blood sugar.

GETTING FAMILIAR WITH YOUR GIANT FOOD LIST

You will find many familiar foods on the Giant Food List. You will also find foods that are more desirable for keeping your chemistry under control and others that are less desirable and should be avoided or indulged in sparingly. A quick and easy guide to direct how you select foods, the Giant Food List is divided into three general categories of foods:

Pure Power: These foods provide the most power (nutrients) with the least amount of punch (trigger potential for the Metabolic Mix-Up). High quality proteins and low-starch veggies produce a minimal insulin response and will not challenge your blood sugar balance.

Middle Road: These foods give you good nutrition with a moderate degree of reaction potential. The veggies are more starchy, the proteins more fatty, and the fruits more sweet. They will trigger you if you're not careful, so approach the Middle Road with wisdom.

Lower Rung: These foods offer you limited nutrition with the greatest degree of insulin reaction. You will find the most starchy of carbs on this list, as well as the most fat-laden desserts and proteins. If I were including junk food and other processed foods (which I'm not because I think you know these by heart) on the Giant Food List, this is where they'd fall, in the Lower Rung.

You will feel much more energy when you eat as many foods from the Pure Power list as possible, judiciously allowing in some of the healthier starchy carbs from the Middle Road list. You will be safe from the risk of triggering your insulin insult, you will be delivering lasting nutrition to your body and brain, and you will enable your body to metabolize the foods you eat most efficiently.

PICK YOUR FRIENDS WISELY

Carbohydrates can be broken down into three simple sugars, so choose carefully.

- Glucose is absorbed by the body the most quickly and therefore releases the most intense call for insulin. Foods such as starches, grains, and sugars break down into glucose.
- Galactose is the by-product of dairy products and has a slower uptake by the body because it needs to be converted into glucose before it calls for the insulin.
- Fructose has the slowest absorption rate because it is converted into glucose by the liver.

You may, however, be tempted by the other foods on the Middle Road list. You may choose from this list, just don't use it to plan your entire day's menu. Be sure to include plenty from Pure Power. The Lower Rung stands alone. These foods may be satisfying in the short term, but they also will invite your chemistry to overreact. Remember that your chemistry works in predictable ways. The foods you eat today will affect how you feel tomorrow, and what you eat in the morning will affect how you feel in the evening. The more foods you eat from the Pure Power group, the better you will feel—today, tomorrow, and the days after that.

But I am also realistic. You can live your *real* life, choosing some of the less desirable foods from the Middle Road and occasionally from the Lower Rung, and at the same time sustain your sense of well-being. To ensure that you manage your mix-up while eating these less desirable foods, you will learn certain techniques—such as increasing supplements or exercise—in order to minimize your reactions by maximizing your metabolism. Some of the foods on the Lower Rung list may be better for your soul than for your chemistry, so just *be reasonable*. Eat these foods only when it seems to be important and you're feeling really balanced, ready to take on the challenge that will inevitably come, making adjustments along the way.

GOOD FOR YOUR SOUL

Birthday cake on your birthday may not be good for your body, but it sure is good for your soul. Allowing yourself to have an occasional trigger food (a simple carb) that you love is as important for your health as keeping in better balance the rest of the time.

THE PURE-POWER PROMISE

The more foods you choose from the Pure Power list, the more likely you can:

- Lessen your craving
- Strengthen your concentration
- Increase your energy level
- Lose weight
- Heighten your attention span
- Feel more serene and balanced
- Reduce your BMI
- Create more muscle and lessen fat to better your body composition
- Reduce cholesterol, triglycerides, and blood pressure

And all of these together tell you that you are taming your Metabolic Mix-Up and reducing your risk of more serious disease.

THE REASONABLE RANGE FOR PORTION SIZES AND AMOUNTS

It may still be hard for you not to think about calories, ounces, or grams; and that is no surprise. We have just begun to work toward creating a new style of eating that feels cozy and right. Once you are in balanced blood sugar, you will become very reliable, no longer responding to that misleading impulse that tells you to eat the wrong things at the wrong times. You will also be more likely to choose to eat a *reasonable* amount of food for you.

I don't want you to be sitting with spoons and cups and scales, getting bogged down by measuring your foods. Once you become familiar with these easy instructions, you will be able to eyeball reasonable amounts as naturally as you move through the steps.

What is a reasonable range? There are four rules that apply, depending on whether you're eating a starchy carbohydrate, a protein (fish, meat, or poultry), or a portion of veggies. (Again, veggies are carbohydrates, but since most are high in fiber and are naturally unrefined, I treat them in their own special category.) Take a look at the hand measurement guide below.

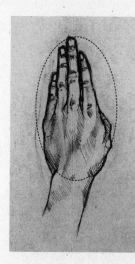

EXTENDED HAND:
Hand held out, palm down, fingers extended, thumb folded in. This is the reasonable amount for a fish fillet.

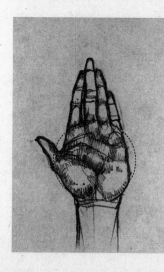

OPEN PALM:
Palm facing up. Do not count the fingers, just the palm. This is the reasonable amount for meat or poultry.

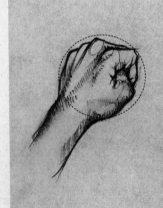

CLOSED FIST:
Place your fist flat on a table, with the thumb folded in. This is the reasonable amount for a starchy carb portion.

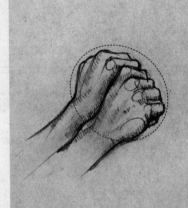

CLOSED DOUBLE FIST:
Place both fists flat on a table, with both thumbs folded in. This is the *minimum* amount of veggies and/or salad!

These hand measurements are general approximations of reasonable amounts, depending on your physical size, whether you are a man or a woman, or how much weight you may want to lose.

Another way to accomplish the reasonable range for portion sizes and amounts is by picturing a plate and dividing it so that one-fourth of it is made up of nutrient-laden carbohydrates and the rest is made up of veggies and high-quality protein. However, if you are not having a starchy carbohydrate, then divide your plate between one-third protein and two-thirds veggies. A little more or a little less is okay, too.

That's it. End of story.

Not so difficult and not so exotic. Don't make things more complicated than they need to be. I know you have lived with the dieter's dilemma for a long time (how much is too much?), but you are traveling a new road to health that begins and ends with controlling your chemistry. Once you do this, vibrant health will follow whether or not you want to lose or maintain weight.

If you're wondering about how much swordfish to eat or how much spinach goes on your plate, just use your reasonable range hand guide, and don't worry if your hand size offers you a slightly larger amount of food. Being reasonable is the goal. The size of your hand is most likely in line with the size of your body, offering more for larger and less for petite. You will require a different amount of food considering whether you are a man or woman; have a big, medium, or small frame; exercise seven days a week or three or not at all; or take supplements. As you will learn in the next few chapters, you can eat most veggies to your heart's content. Be more moderate with those vegetables that fall in the Middle Road list. Those you should eat more sparingly and more judiciously. And the Lower Rung list as well, beware!

American restaurants are notorious for using huge amounts to market to customers: Don't be fooled. You do not get more for your money when you are served a plate overflowing with food.

You are merely training your body and eye to expect these over-sized and unnecessary portions.

In France, where nearly everyone is thin and the average cholesterol level is much lower than that of the average American, you may have a three-course meal at a restaurant, but note that the serving sizes are small. If you order chicken, you may get a breast or a leg, but you won't get both. Do the French (or will you) walk away feeling hungry? No, because you're eating enough of the right food to satisfy your body. My point? Don't get distracted by amounts, just be reasonable, and perhaps a bit European in mind.

THE FRENCH PARADOX

Although we would love to believe that frequent consumption of red wine is solely responsible for the low cholesterol of the French people, it is *also* their concept of what constitutes an appropriate meal.

IT'S ALL IN THE TIMING

After a night's sleep, everyone wakes up in unbalanced or low blood sugar. This is normal. Your body has used up its energy reserve and needs to refuel. If you stay in low blood sugar, you can be spacey, forgetful, anxious, and crave starches, sweets, alcohol, caffeine, or fats. This is true for everyone in lesser to higher degrees of intensity. However, when you have the Metabolic Mix-Up, this need to refuel is even more critical because we are more sensitive to *any* imbalance in blood sugar. The timing of a healthy morning breakfast and a midmorning snack is crucial to controlling your chemistry right away.

Controlling your insulin resistance not only requires that you are reasonable in both your selection of foods and their amounts but it also requires that you eat at regular intervals through-out the day. If you follow your old eat-when-you-feel-like-it or when-somebody-else-feels-like-it routine, you will stay where you've been all along—down and out. Now some of you may not know that you feel less than you can. When you pay atten-tion to the timing of foods, you take the first step in making sure that your brain is delivered its critical fuel. The brain relies on glucose to perform and it can't store any. The minute you get into low blood sugar, you literally alter your brain activity. Like a finicky infant, your brain needs food at regular intervals to live. And when you give it food at regular times, in reasonable amounts, and in the highest quality, it will function at its very best. And any alteration in brain chemistry means an alteration in how you feel. Remember how when your blood sugar is out of balance you can feel anxious or depressed and become more vulnerable to mood swings? It is the brain that gives your body the signal of how to feel. If you feed it as you would a beloved dinner guest it will send a thank-you, telling your body to feel remarkable. If you feed the brain carelessly, then it's more likely you will be punished than thanked. It's that simple.

On the Carb-Careful Solution you eat three meals a day with at least one snack in the morning (between breakfast and lunch) and one in the afternoon (between lunch and dinner).

Eating in this way also helps you to avoid triggering your in-sulin resistance. It will affect how you feel tomorrow and the day after tomorrow. Soon you will experience a glorious sense of satisfaction in how much you can accomplish in any given day.

TAPPING INTO THE MIRACLE OF WATER

You're probably tired of hearing that you should drink eight glasses of water a day. Most of us are. But water is an essential part of a healthy diet because it has so many purposes, and the news is that you really need a minimum of ten glasses a day, and that's if it's not hot or you're not working out. How do you know if you are drinking enough water? Try pinching your skin. If your skin remains puckered for any length of time, then you are probably dehydrated. Dehydration—even the mildest—can take a toll on your body. And by the time you wait to feel thirsty, you are already dehydrated. Recently during a hot spell, my husband and I went out to dinner with my usually bubbly and vibrant mother-in-law. She seemed quiet and pale, a clear sign that she wasn't feeling well. When I noticed that she had barely touched her favorite dish, I asked her if she was feeling okay. She said that she was feeling "fine, just a bit fuzzy." She looked anything but fine. I then asked her a few more questions. It was hard not to, considering that she was looking as though she belonged in bed. When I asked her how much water she'd had during that day, she replied, "Oh plenty! I had plenty."

After returning home, I continued to think about how listless she had been. Concerned about my mother-in-law, I called to ask exactly how much water she'd had that day. I learned a long time ago to get the specifics, realizing that perceptions are unique to each individual. So I was not surprised to hear that her plenty was only three glasses. Clearly not enough! I then instructed her to drink at least three to four glasses of water in the next hour. When I called her back an hour later, I heard the old kick in her voice, much to my relief. Just goes to show you how one person's desert is another person's Niagara Falls.

Water is essential to your body's metabolism. Not only does it help mobilize fat, it also cleanses your body of toxins, which, if left behind, can leave a nasty trail. Like the rest of the Midlife Miracle Diet, once you become more conscious of drinking water—keeping a bottle on your desk as you work, taking a bottle with you in the car, drinking a glass when you wake up and when you go to bed—then you will miss it when you don't drink enough and that will be reminder enough. Again, try to drink at least ten glasses a day—that's a minimum requirement. However, a more precise way to figure out how much water you should be drinking is to use the following formula: 1 ounce of water per every 2 pounds of body weight. So if you weigh 200 pounds, you should be drinking 112.5 ounces of water—that's about fourteen 8-ounce glasses of water. If you weigh 155 pounds, you should be drinking at least 77.5 ounces, or almost ten glasses of water.

YOU ALWAYS NEED PLENTY OF WATER

In addition to your ten to twelve daily glasses of water, remember to increase your water intake:

- If you exercise
- In hot weather
- When you are sick or feverish
- During weight loss

YOUR JOURNAL KEEPS YOU CONSCIOUS

Keep a journal recording the foods you eat and when you eat them. You can use any kind of notebook you like. By writing down the foods you eat at each meal or snack, you are paying attention to what you are eating. It doesn't mean you won't slip up. It simply means that you are committing to staying present and to making a specific attempt to eat differently and to deal with these changes. The journal enables you to be real. It allows you to know how you are really doing so that you are not surprised or dismayed by how you feel. Instead of deluding yourself into thinking you deserve the Bronze Star for good behavior when you have really just devoured a bag of chips, your journal will keep you conscious.

How can a journal be so important? I find that people who write are more likely to stay present and accountable each and every day as they become familiar with this new style of eating. Life can leave you stressed and distracted, and the journal will help you remember what you are trying to do. Know that it will help you feel more prepared to deal with challenges along the way. When you can relate to the everyday impact of the foods on your emotional ups and downs, you will no longer choose a food style that makes you feel like you're riding up the down escalator. Some people don't keep the journal because they don't want to know what they have done, or they feel bad or wish to escape—without even letting themselves know they have declared food freedom by allowing themselves mindlessly to eat whatever comes their way.

Take a look at the sample journal entries in the Appendix. You can see how my clients use the journal to keep track and keep aware of what they eat and when they eat. You will also find a blank journal page that you can use as a model. But feel free to keep a record of your foods in whatever form that works for you.

THE TALE OF TWO GLYCEMIC INDEXES

Remember how those of us with the Metabolic Mix-Up have to move our belt buckles after eating a bag of popcorn or a bagel? Or how once you have one cookie, you find yourself inhaling the entire box? This is because the glycemic index (GI) of these starchy, sugary delights is high, and foods with a high glycemic response, such as white and brown sugar, honey, fruit juices, and starchy carbohydrates (breads, pastas, cereals, white rice, white potatoes, and corn) cause a rapid rise in insulin levels. You may not have connected how you feel to what you eat, but these foods with a high GI are a primary reason you get heady and feel more tired so quickly after eating starchy and sugary foods.

But though the GI looks on the surface to be a surefire way to select foods that won't trigger your mix-up, the GI itself is under full investigation by many research groups because people's responses to foods vary so much. These are just a few of the factors involved:

- The same food eaten at different times of day in different combinations will produce a different reaction.
- The preparation of the food can change the glycemic impact of that food.
- The GI response also depends on where the food is grown; different geographical areas contain different nutrients in the soil, altering the character of the food itself.
- Reactions vary from person to person since not everyone has the same chemistry.

There are also two glycemic indexes. In the past, most GIs used glucose to measure the blood sugar response of a particular food. However, since most people asked to test the GI rating of a food did not want to ingest 50 grams of pure glucose (not a tasty proposition), the researchers began using white bread as the standard to rate a food's blood sugar response. People were much more inclined to eat 50 grams of white bread. The result? The GI of most of the foods shifted, and in most cases, foods were recorded as being more highly glycemic than previously reported, causing a lot of confusion.

The GI can be a useful tool in helping to point us in the direction of foods that are less likely to cause an insulin reaction, but your body and its reactions are the most reliable indicator of the trigger factor of a particular food. If you become hungry or begin to crave, or even experience a drop in energy, then the food you recently ate—regardless of its GI rating—is probably too reactive for you.

The three tiers of the Giant Food List take into account the GI of the foods listed. Pure-power foods have the lowest GI ratings; middle-road foods have a moderate GI rating; and lower-rung foods have a high GI rating. Don't be confused; the higher the GI, the more damaging the food. Foods with a lower GI have a slower glycemic response and will not spike insulin levels and therefore will avoid triggering your Metabolic Mix-Up.

CHECK OUT YOUR FRUIT PUNCH

Fruits are not all alike: Those that are highly reactive appear higher on the glycemic index and can trigger your Metabolic Mix-Up; those that are less glycemic (lower on the GI) are easier on your metabolism.

Less reactive fruits: apple, berries, grapefruit, kiwi, nectarine, pear, and plum.

Highly reactive fruits: banana, cantaloupe, cranberries, mango, papaya, raisins, and any fruit that has been dried, mashed, juiced, or soaked in syrup.

CHAPTER 5

Step One: Creating Basic Balance

IT ALL BEGINS WITH BALANCED BLOOD SUGAR

Before you can talk yourself into eating in a new and different way, you have to talk to your chemistry. No matter how much discipline or willpower you may have, no matter how hard you try, you cannot change your body without first controlling your chemistry. This means getting into good blood sugar balance and staying there.

Basic Balance is designed to do just that: This first step of the Carb-Careful Solution helps to balance your blood sugar so that you are no longer craving. You may still be looking for food, but you are no longer longing for it. Based on the need to slow down the call for carbohydrates, Basic Balance prevents the inevitable beginning of the Metabolic Mix-Up undertow. Remember that much of the body's fuel comes from carbohydrates? It's not as if we don't need them; we do. Carbohydrates are essential for health, especially for brain function. But when you have this disorder of metabolism you react to carbohydrates more intensely. Because your insulin resistance is getting in the way of the insulin's ability to penetrate the cells, it becomes impossible for you to benefit from those carbs that you do eat. As a result, you crave more, eat more, and as if that's not bad enough, you trigger the release of more ineffective insulin. When your brain doesn't receive its supply of fuel, you can feel foggy, disoriented, and even forgetful. And to add insult to injury, this unsuccessful insulin as a storage hormone signals the body to become a fat-making machine.

By getting into Basic Balance, you redesign your chemistry so that you don't incite this roller-coaster call for carbs. And once you reduce the amount and pay more careful attention to what you eat and when you eat, you will begin to see some pretty dramatic results. Once you are separated from that almost obsessive connection to those starchy and sweet foods, you will not only be free from craving but you will also start to experience a sense of calm coupled with a powerful vitality.

As Margaret, a very busy mother of five said of Basic Balance, "I feel like a different person! I am no longer crawling through the day—even my family sees the difference. I'm not jumpy anymore. I'm even able to find a decent amount of time to spend with each of my kids." For Margaret and all of us with the Metabolic Mix-Up, the key to her sudden and real shift in mood came with balancing her blood sugar. In Basic Balance, you'll no longer have all those highs and lows, peaks and valleys, where one minute you feel like you could run a marathon or pass up that sweet and the next you are eating the crust of every piece of bread in sight.

The result? You will have more energy than you ever had before. You'll want to take a nice walk, run, or even sign up for that wild spin class that only the brave dare enter. Once you are in Basic Balance, you can improve playing everything from baseball to chess. I've worked with all sorts of men and women—teachers, sports figures, media specialists, researchers, actors, construction workers, and police officers—who have all experienced an increase in stamina, focus, and concentration, which enhances the quality of their lives and allows them to function on a higher level.

Controlling your blood sugar and maintaining it in balance *creates* energy, and you will find this energy literally coursing through your veins. When you feel remarkably better, free at last from the power of foods, you will have arrived and you will know it. You will no longer need me to encourage you; you will be living in your life, feeling the health and the energy every minute. Before getting into Basic Balance, one client of mine, Marly, a jazz performer in Los Angeles, had become accustomed to the quality of her performance depending on which part of the blood sugar roller coaster she was riding. She described the shift in her life in this way, "I'm now able to stay in my power place. I feel lighthearted, excited, and joyful."

DON'T PANIC BECAUSE OF THE BLOOD SUGAR BLUES!

If you trigger your Metabolic Mix-Up and find yourself lethargic, anxious, or depressed and craving sweets, you can be sure your blood sugar has run amok. You may be feeling challenged, but it should help to know the cravings won't last. Just go back to Basic Balance as soon as you can. And know that it will take just forty-eight to seventy-two hours to readjust your body chemistry. Be patient. It's worth the wait!

HOW TO BEGIN BASIC BALANCE: AT A GLANCE

Here comes our refrain: Balanced blood sugar is key not only in managing your insulin resistance, giving you wonderful energy and a greater sense of well-being but also in giving you the ability to lose weight and keep it off if that's what you want to do. Basic Balance does all this for you, and more. By following the simple instructions, you will begin the shift from mediocre health to a level of magnificent health that you may not have ever believed was possible—all because you are beginning to tame that menacing Metabolic Mix-Up.

Remember that timing, placement, and reasonable amounts of foods are all crucial to creating Basic Balance. All of these tools that you've learned earlier come into play here. Here's a quick recap:

- Use your Giant Food List to select the most pure-power foods as possible, adding some middle-road choices as you go.
- Put together a plate that is a nutritious combination of foods in reasonable amounts.
- Time meals and snacks so that you eat three meals a day and at least two snacks at regular intervals that match your particular schedule.
- Drink plenty of water to keep your body hydrated.
- Keep a record of your foods in your journal.

When you are in Basic Balance, the food will not have to be glamorous. Oh yes, sometimes it will be glorious—for celebrations, on holidays, at really great restaurants—but for the most part, you will eat to feel well and go on with your day. You will no longer feel seduced by foods that trigger you. Instead, food that used to be your foe will become your friend. Basic Balance will free you from the power of your cravings and give you such peace of mind that you will never again have to worry about being vulnerable to an emotional roller coaster caused by imbalanced blood sugar.

Read through the typical day described below. This overview will give you a good general idea of how and when to eat. Don't be alarmed if I don't mention your favorite food right away; you will find an abundant list of foods from which to choose in your Giant Food List and from the menus at the end of this chapter.

Breakfast

As Mama used to say, breakfast is the most important meal of the day. Well, this is partially true. It's definitely the *first* most important meal of the day. What we eat for breakfast usually depends an awful lot on how we were brought up, what we ate the night before, and what we hear on the late night news. In my house, the first thing staring at me in the morning was corn flakes *with sugar,* a piece of French Toast *with sugar,* or a bagel and peanut butter, also *with sugar.* These combinations propelled me out of the house and over to school, but once there, I would begin my inevitable nosedive into no energy. Genetically and environmentally programmed to have the Metabolic Mix-Up, this rapid release of sugar into the bloodstream orchestrated each day to begin with an uphill battle, always resulting in an out of control ride on a downhill course in my blood sugar cart. An hour or so later, I would be craving the sugar I so badly needed.

The power of your chemistry is too strong to ignore. Unless you begin the day in the right way, you will continue to be a slave to a constant intake of carbs and sugar, addicted to satisfying your craving. When you start the morning by eating a breakfast of pure power, then you'll be in balanced blood sugar by noon, in charge of your choices, and in control of your cravings.

How to Eat

• **It's essential to eat breakfast soon after you wake up.** Try to eat within the first hour or so. The reason for this is simple: We all wake up in a state of low blood sugar. But if you stay in this wake-up state, you will crave for the rest of the day. Begin your Basic Balance as soon as possible by eating something satisfying from the Giant Food List.

• **Yes, yes, you can have a cup of coffee.** If you must, just forget the sugar, and decaf is preferred. In the future you won't even need this pick-me-up! And remember to start drinking your water. If you want to lose weight, you may also want to skip the half-and-half—use low-fat milk or try some plain soy milk instead.

• **Your breakfast needs to contain a protein.** This is very important, so please do not forget to include it. Unlike the bagels and other starches, which quickly break down into glucose and put your body into overdrive, protein acts to slow down the release, providing your body with ongoing vital fuel to begin the day.

• **You can eat a starch with breakfast.** We are addicted to eating breads and cereals at the beginning of the day. But if you do have cereal, forget the fruit. And if you really need to have that onion bagel, be sure to add a protein such as soy cheese or a dollop of unsweetened peanut butter. By adding the protein to the carbohydrate, you will protect your body from being slammed with insulin, giving it more than it can handle, and getting you off to a less than wonderful start. And always remember when you're selecting a protein, choose one that is high quality, one that is low in fat and salt.

• **Try veggies with breakfast.** Did you eat veggies last night for dinner? Why not have the leftover veggies with your protein for breakfast. These pure-power carbs are a great way to start the day. Leftover grilled or stir-fried veggies are a great alternative.

• **If you want to be more original,** go outside your typical breakfast foods and try proteins such as fish, poultry, or meat. For those of you who have dined in Europe, where it is often customary to eat meat and fish for breakfast, you may feel more inclined to expand your morning repertoire.

• **Alternate cereal and bread.** If you like cereal for breakfast, make sure you don't combine it with bread. Otherwise, you will trigger too much of a blood sugar response early in the day.

• **If you are still dreaming of a starchy carb breakfast, such as waffles or pancakes,** that's okay. We are only at the first step. Just keep it to every other day at the most, switch to whole-grain waffles, and skip the syrup.

What to Eat for Breakfast

Please note that what follows is a list of menu suggestions for what to eat for breakfast; it's by no means a complete list of foods. Consult the Giant Food List (pages 93–103) as well as the menus at the end of this chapter for other meal ideas.

STARCH:
   whole-grain bread, such as rye, whole wheat, or seven-grain
   rye crackers
   brown rice crackers
   less desirable but amenable: white breads, biscuits, croissants

PROTEIN:
   egg whites (use organic when available)
   whole eggs

tofu

non- or low-fat cottage cheese

low- or nonfat cheese

soy cheese (This comes in many varieties, including American, Swiss, mozzarella, and jalapeno. Individually wrapped stays fresh longer.)

almond or peanut butter (unsweetened) (Limit nut butters as they tend to be high in fat and sodium.)

poultry or fish

CEREAL PLUS LOW-FAT MILK:

bran flakes

cream of rice

cream of wheat

kashi

oatmeal

shredded wheat

other totally unsweetened cereals

THE DANGER OF THE DILLYDALLY BREAKFAST

It's important to be aware of *when* you eat breakfast. Perhaps you're like Anna, who is in the habit of waking up leisurely at about eight or nine o'clock and lingering over her coffee for an hour as she reads the paper and watches a bit of the morning news. After forty-five minutes, she usually eats a frozen waffle with syrup. By this time it's only ten-thirty and she's managed to send her body into a biochemical tailspin. If you start your day like Anna by waiting to eat a breakfast loaded with starchy, refined carbohydrates and sugar, you are looking for trouble. By immediately starting the cycle of high and then low blood sugar, you will create the cycle of carb craving and set into motion the damages engineered by your Metabolic Mix-Up—your insulin resistance and hyperinsulinemia.

Morning Snacks

A healthy breakfast deserves a healthy morning snack. After a few days, you'll be surprised at how good you feel as you start your day. Everyone is. You'll feel clearheaded and raring to go, returning those phone calls or finishing those errands in record time. Simply remember to continue having your morning snack. Once you start feeling better and less needy, it's easy to forget to have them. Don't think you can. In order to hold on to the good feelings, you need to hold on to your snacks.

How to Eat

• **Do not wait until lunch to eat again.** It's imperative that you snack at least once between breakfast and lunch.

• **If you eat breakfast early, then you need a second snack before lunchtime.** You need to refuel yourself at regular intervals without going too long without food. Snacking this way helps you achieve a more balanced blood sugar level by lunchtime, even if that means you'll eat again in one hour for lunch. My schedule includes two morning snacks because I eat breakfast so early (at around 6:30 A.M.); I eat my first snack at 8:30 A.M. and my next at around 10:30 A.M.

• **Don't randomly nibble at your snack all morning.** Just a warning, but this kind of eating will actually hinder your goal of balancing your blood sugar by lunchtime. If you have bits and pieces over a long period of time, you never quite have quite enough to be in Basic Balance, and you are continually challenging your system. You need to eat at regular, two- to three-hour intervals—the right amount of glucose at the right time to balance your blood sugar.

• **Hard Chew snacks are the best to choose from.** What exactly are these? Any raw vegetable or raw fruit that is essentially hard to chew. Pretty much what you would imagine: celery stalks, carrots, apples, or any of the other numerous Hard Chew veggies or fruits that you have seen in the marketplace—or in the fields. These snacks should be raw, unprocessed and uncooked. The less cooked they are, the less insulin they will call for. The cooking actually changes the chemical makeup of the vegetable by breaking down the fiber, making the glucose available for quick release.

What to Eat

Here is a sampling of Hard Chews:

apple
asparagus stalks
broccoli
carrots
cauliflower
celery stalks
daikon radish chunks
fennel bulbs
Kirby cucumber
pear
red cabbage chunks
string beans

WHAT IS A KIRBY?

A small, crisp delicious cucumber used for pickling, unpickled of course.

HOLD ON TO THE GOOD FEELINGS

Just when people start to feel terrific, they often forget how they got that way. The program is magic, but you didn't arrive at feeling so weak by waving a stick over your head. Don't forget to continue Basic Balance to ensure your sense of well-being.

A WARNING FOR SENSITIVE STOMACHS

For some people who have colitis or an ulcer, eating Hard Chews—like too many raw veggies and fruit—can be a problem because of that condition. In this case, be sure to blanch, slightly steam, or microwave your veggies to the point that they will not challenge your digestive system.

Lunch

Most of us, like the children we once were, look forward to the break in the day that lunchtime will bring. You should feel balanced, at ease, and interested and ready to eat, but not starving. By the time you finish your midday meal, you will be feeling the wonderful effects of eating right all morning.

How to Eat
• **It's best if you can eat your second meal by 1 P.M.** Your body needs a midday meal to maintain the balance you've introduced in the morning.
• **Lunch should be made up mostly of protein and veggies.**
• **You can include a starch; an unrefined complex carb is best,** but try to choose one from the pure-power or middle-road list on the Giant Food List.
• **Don't forget the Hard Chew veggie at lunch.** A small amount added to your salad is all you need. The Hard Chews are just another ingredient that helps lock blood sugar into place.
• **Basta pasta.** The only carbohydrate that is definitely *not* allowed at lunch is pasta. This will just give you a quick-carb fix and leave you craving for more in no time. The pasta you love does not love you. It will literally dissolve your blood sugar serenity by immediately releasing a call for insulin—a sure way to trigger your Metabolic Mix-Up. I'm reminding you because

it's easy to forget. If you ask someone for an example of a carbohydrate, nine times out of ten he'll say pasta.

• **Give veggies a major role.** Meals that star protein and starch and relegate veggies to a minor role are unhealthy and undermine blood sugar balance.

• **Veggie delight! You can eat any nonstarchy vegetable to your heart's content**—raw, steamed, stir-fried, or grilled. Just remember: Watch the amount of oil you use. Be creative. Look at the Giant Food List for the best pure-power or middle-road vegetable choices. There are wonderful cookbooks whose main focus is preparing and cooking vegetables with recipes that tweak the palate.

HARD CHEW GRAB BAG

Sometimes when I am short of time, I will cut any variety of high-fiber veggies and place them all in the same plastic bag. During the day, I can then dip into the bag and come out with a handful of my favorite veggies. Cauliflower, radishes, fennel, and string beans seem to be the ones I most often mix. But don't stop there. Let your taste buds and your imagination run wild.

What to Eat

Remember these meal suggestions are meant to spark menu ideas; by no means is this a complete listing of foods you can enjoy for lunch.

PROTEIN:
   chicken, turkey, fish
   lean deli meats such as turkey and ham
   nonfat cheese

low-fat cottage cheese
soy cheese
tofu
lean beef, lamb, or veal
egg whites
vegetarian substitute meats with no more than 5 grams carbohydrates

---

REMEMBER YOUR GIANT FOOD LIST

You will find lots of your favorite foods on the Giant Food List at
the end of this chapter.

VEGGIES:

Almost any nonstarchy veggies that are grilled, steamed, stir-
fried, or raw:

  Grilled—eggplant, fennel, radicchio
  Lightly marinated—broccoli rabe, mushrooms
  Raw—cherry tomatoes, celery
  Salad—all kinds of lettuce
  Steamed—asparagus, brussels sprouts
  Stir-fried—onions, carrots, broccoli, spinach

STARCH:

★**Warning.** If you suspect you are carb sensitive—and you probably are if you are reading this book—do not add a starch at
lunch if you have not already been having them.

  baked potato
  bean or lentil soup
  brown rice

pita pocket or bread
yam

THE PASTA YOU LOVE

You have an enormous list of great, delicious carbs to choose from for lunch—but not pasta! You know that after-lunch slump? The time you'd rather be anywhere but where you are and back in bed is beginning to sound good? That's what happens if you eat pasta at lunch. It will dissolve your blood sugar serenity, leaving you craving and exhausted.

Afternoon Snacks

Your afternoon snacks are just as important as your morning snack for keeping you in Basic Balance. Don't be seduced into skipping your food because you are busy and feeling so satisfied. Remember what you eat today will impact how you feel tomorrow. It's almost the end of the day and you're doing so well.

How to Eat
• **Choose a Hard Chew veggie.** The hard chew veggies are better for helping balance your blood sugar because they contain fiber, which takes longer to digest and therefore goes more slowly into your bloodstream.

• **You can also have a Hard *or* soft Chew fruit.** The soft chews release sugar into your body's cells more quickly than Hard Chews, working more like a quick-fix sweet, so we save them for the afternoon when your body is in well-balanced blood sugar and much less susceptible to overreacting to a too-big insulin release.

• **Soft Chew fruit will help you head off that cry for sugar.** And it's still much better than an Oreo cookie. If in need, scoop yourself some extra berries before you reach for the cookie jar.

• **And because you are in Basic Balance, you can go longer between snacks.** Perhaps have your first afternoon snack several hours after your lunch.

• **You'll need to have another late afternoon snack after this initial one if you are eating late.** It's the timing that is important; you should be eating something regularly every few hours.

What to Eat

HARD CHEW VEGGIES
  cucumbers
  green beans
  broccolini
  red cabbage

SOFT CHEW SNACKS
  cantaloupe
  clementine
  grapefruit
  nectarine
  orange
  peach
  plum
  strawberries

WRITE IT DOWN!

Don't forget to write down your meals and snacks in your journal. You can even use your journal to plan your meals ahead of time. The journal is your private coach, helping you to review your moves while reminding you to pay attention as you walk the steps.

Dinner

For many of us, dinner is the main meal of the day, and we like it to be our most important. I know in my family it certainly was when I was growing up. And for my husband and me, it still is since it is our time to be together. However, it is no longer necessary to eat a lot. My clients agree that dinner doesn't need to be the main event that it used to be since they've begun to arrive at the table in Basic Balance.

How to Eat

• **What is dinner?** Basically the same as lunch: your choice of protein and veggie, and a starchy carbohydrate if you would like and have not had one for lunch.

• **The last part of dinner, the starchy carbohydrate, is optional.** If weight is an issue, then only have it for lunch *or* dinner on alternating days.

• **If you're going to have pasta, now is the time.** If you've been in good blood sugar all day, you can add a tomato sauce to your pasta and still manage to avoid triggering a huge call for insulin. Be modest in your selection of sauce and eliminate thick, sweetened ones. Travel to Italy by spicing up your pasta with a flavored olive oil or chicken broth instead.

• **If you'd like a vegetarian meal, dinner is a good time to have it.** Just be sure to include a starchy carb from your purepower or middle-road list, and don't forget your veggies and protein. You would be surprised to learn how many vegetarians drape themselves in starches, leaving the bulk of their veggies back in the garden.

What to Eat

PROTEIN
  poultry or fish
  soy cheese
  tofu or tempeh

nonfat cheese

beef, lamb, veal or pork (though
keep these foods to twice a
week at the most because of
their fat content)

VEGGIES

Again, you can have almost any.
Slice them, dice them but be sure
to include them.

STARCHES

NOTE: *If you had a starch for lunch,
then skip it for dinner.*

baked potato

brown or white rice

couscous

pasta (remember, twice a week at
the maximum)

beans or bean soup

lentils

peas or corn, acorn or butternut squash (while these are veggies, you will see when you consult your Giant Food List
that they are more starchy and fall into middle-road and
lower-rung categories, so they should be eaten in moderation)

> **MEAT AND
> POTATOES WILL
> NO LONGER BE
> AS TEMPTING**
>
> When you're doing
> Basic Balance, you will
> be much less at-
> tracted to starchy car-
> bohydrates and fatty
> proteins, such as meat
> and potatoes. So get
> into Basic Balance
> and those french fries
> and burgers will no
> longer be calling your
> name.

> ## ALL PASTAS ARE NOT ALIKE
>
> The trigger potential of pastas depends on four factors:
>
> 1. The amount of protein in the pasta: the more protein, the less reactive
> 2. The other ingredients in the pasta: the more fat and fiber included, the less reactive
> 3. The length of cooking time: the more al dente, the less reactive
> 4. The shape and density of the pasta itself: the harder the pasta, the less reactive
>
> So the next time you want to indulge in some pasta, choose penne over fettucine, macaroni over lasagne.

SAMPLE MENUS

These menus are meant to be suggestions to add spice and spirit to your meals. Use the times as guidelines, adjusting your eating schedule to when you wake up and eat breakfast, lunch, and dinner. Notice how a second afternoon snack is added when your dinner is later than 7:00 P.M. Never go more than three hours without eating a snack or a meal or else you will interrupt that beautiful Basic Balance. Don't worry about including the suggested carbohydrates in this step. You'll notice I did not include beverage suggestions in the menus. I'll leave this up to your best judgment (and the Giant Food List), but please be sure to drink plenty of water, water, water! Enjoy!

Day One

Breakfast: (7:30 A.M.) Egg-white burrito in whole-wheat tortilla, with chopped tomatoes

Snack: (9:30 A.M.) Baby carrots

Snack: (11:30 A.M.)	Healthy handful of string beans
Lunch: (12:30 P.M.)	Discreet chef's salad: Large chopped salad with sliced turkey as only deli meat. Sprinkle with balsamic vinegar and a dash of olive oil. Add celery in salad as your Hard Chew.
Snack: (3:30 P.M.)	1 orange
Dinner: (6:00 P.M.)	Chinese takeout with brown rice and steamed vegetables. Include some tofu for protein.

⋆REMINDER: *When you have more than one complex carb . . . and you find yourself craving, then begin to monitor yourself more closely.*

Day Two

Breakfast: (7:00 A.M.)	Small portion of low- or nonfat hard cheese Piece of eight-grain bread
Snack: (9:00 A.M.)	Plain yogurt (sugar-free and fat-free) with raw apple
Snack: (11:00 A.M.)	Healthy handful of celery
Lunch: (12:30 P.M.)	Whole-wheat pita pocket with lean ham, mustard, and tomato with two radishes
Snack: (3:30 P.M.)	1 peach or nectarine
Dinner: (7:00 P.M.)	Steamed lobster with garlic black bean sauce (made without sugar), side of sauteed spinach, and green salad with cut-up endive

Day Three

Breakfast: (7:30 A.M.)	Bowl muesli (unsweetened) with 1% milk and without fruit
Snack: (10:30 A.M.)	1 apple
Lunch: (1:00 P.M.)	Grilled vegetables brushed sparingly with olive oil, and reasonable portion grilled chicken.
Snack: (4:00 P.M.)	Nectarine
Dinner: (8:00 P.M.)	Black beans simmered with onions, garlic, pepper, and cilantro
	Grey sole steamed with lemon
	Mixed greens with balsamic vinegar
	Broccoli with garlic and olive oil

Day Four

Breakfast: (7:00 A.M.)	Whole-grain bread, toasted and spread with unsweetened peanut butter
Snack: (9:30 A.M.)	Baby carrots
Snack: (11:00 A.M.)	1 apple
Lunch: (12:30 P.M.)	Grilled shrimp
	Steamed mixed vegetables
	Whole radishes (Remember, your hard chew is important at lunch.)
Snack: (3:00 P.M.)	Reasonable amount of Strawberries with low-fat cottage cheese

Dinner: (6:00 P.M.)   Couscous

Broiled lamb chops

Steamed zucchini or asparagus

Mixed green salad with dash of vinaigrette dressing

Day Five

Breakfast: (6:30 A.M.)   Slow-cooked oatmeal with cinnamon

Snack: (9:00 A.M.)   Fennel chunks

Snack: (10:30 A.M.)   Daikon radish

Lunch: (1:00 P.M.)   Mini whole-wheat pita stuffed with tuna salad, chopped red pepper and celery, sprinkled with wine vinegar and green olives (Add a side of crudités: carrot sticks, cucumber slices, and cherry tomatoes.)

Snack: (3:00 P.M.)   Orange

Snack: (5:00 P.M.)   Nectarine

Dinner: (8:00 P.M.)   Spinach and mushroom salad

Roasted chicken, seasoned with herbs de Provence

Steamed cauliflower with grated Parmesan cheese

TRANSFORM AN ORDINARY DISH INTO EXTRAORDINARY

Use herbs de Provence, a flavorful blend of spices that give a hearty taste to meats, tuna steaks, and foods cooked with cabbage, broccoli, garlic, and onions.

Use fines herbes, a gentle herbal blend containing sweet basil, tarragon, and shallots that adds a sweet flavor to soft foods, such as yellow summer squash, carrots, sea bass, lemon sole, and chicken.

Your Giant Food List is your comprehensive guide to choosing foods. As you become familiar with the foods in the three different levels—pure power, middle road, and lower rung—you will feel more confident in choosing the best foods for you.

THE GIANT FOOD LIST

Pure Power

These foods have the highest degree of nutrients with the least capability of triggering your Metabolic Mix-Up.

Proteins

FISH
 bass
 bluefish
 catfish
 cod
 flounder
 grouper
 haddock

halibut
herring
monkfish
pike
pompano
rainbow trout
salmon
sole
swordfish
tilefish
tuna

SHELLFISH
clams
crabmeat
crayfish
lobster
mussels
oysters

MEATS AND POULTRY
Canadian bacon
chicken breasts (skinless)
Cornish hen (skinless)
lamb shank
round steak
sirloin
turkey breast (white meat)
turkey and chicken deli meat (lean)

DAIRY
egg whites
low-fat cottage cheese

VEGETARIAN CHOICES
meat substitutes with 5% or less carbohydrate grams
soy burgers

soy cheese
soy hot dog or sausage
tofu

Carbohydrates

VEGGIES
artichokes
arugula
asparagus
avocado
bok choy
broccoli
brussels sprouts
cabbage
cauliflower
celery
chicory
chinese pea pods
collard greens
cucumbers
daikon (Japanese radishes)
dandelion greens
eggplant
endive
escarole
green beans
Jerusalem artichokes
jicama
kale
kirbys (cucumbers)
kohlrabi
leeks
lettuce (bibb, Boston, green or red leaf, iceberg, romaine)
mushrooms
mustard greens

okra
onions
parsley
peppers (red, green, yellow, or purple)
radishes
scallions
spinach
summer squash
Swiss chard
water chestnuts
zucchini

FRUITS
apple
blueberries
grapefruit
kiwi
lemon
lime
pear
plum

STARCHY CARBS
barley
buckwheat kasha
lentils
oatmeal, slow-cooking
peanuts
soy beans

Condiments

all mustards except honey mustard
all spices and herbs
canola oil

cold-pressed olive oil
olives
vegetable and nonfat chicken broth

Beverages

decaffeinated coffee
decaffeinated herbal teas
herbal teas
seltzer (plain or flavored)
water

Middle Road

These foods provide a good source of nutrients, but some may be either higher in fat, or the carbohydrates are more refined and more starchy; therefore making you more vulnerable to triggering your Metabolic Mix-Up.

Proteins

MEAT AND POULTRY
duck
ground beef (hamburger, lean)
lamb chop (loin or shank, lean or trimmed)
pork (loin or tenderloin, lean or trimmed)
roast beef
turkey (dark meat)
veal (ground or lean)

DAIRY
eggs
mozzarella cheese
ricotta cheese
Danish havarti (light)

REDUCE THESE FATS TO COOK

- butter
- lard or shortening
- margarine
- mixed vegetable oil
- safflower oil
- sesame oil

  Instead, rely on low-fat alternatives when you cook:

- low-salt chicken broth
- olive or canola (flaxseed oil becomes rancid when heated)
- vegetable broth

Carbohydrates

VEGGIES
beets
butternut squash
dried peas
hummus (chick peas)
sauerkraut
sweet potato
tomato
yam

FRUITS
blackberries
boysenberries
cherries
grapes
honeydew melon
nectarine
orange

peach
plantain
raspberries
strawberries
tangelo
tangerine

STARCHY CARBS, LEGUMES AND GRAINS
barley
beans (black beans, kidney beans, lima and pinto beans)
brown rice
bulgur
couscous
mixed grain bread (12- or 9-grain bread)
pumpernickel bread
quinoa
rye bread
rye crackers
wheat germ

Condiments

butter
Italian or caesar dressing
margarine
mayonnaise (in moderation; preferably made with canola oil)

Beverages

milk (1–2% low-fat)
fruit juice

Lower Rung

These foods are your least preferable choices because of their ability to trigger your Metabolic Mix-Up and make you more vulnerable to cravings.

NOTE: Foods that are marked with an asterisk (*) are high in saturated fat and therefore appear on the Lower Rung.

Proteins

MEATS AND POULTRY
  *bacon
  *beef stew or pot roast
  *beef tenderloin
  *corned beef
  *deli meats (bologna, pastrami, salami)
  *ground beef
  *hot dog (beef)
  *kielbasa

NUTS

Nuts are a wonderful snack and a great way to help maintain balanced blood sugar. But they're also easy to overeat, so be careful that you have only a small portion since their high fat content makes them a high calorie trap.

almonds
flaxseeds
hazelnuts
peanuts
pecans
pistachio
pumpkin seeds
sesame seeds
soy nuts
sunflower seeds
walnuts

---

*liver (beef or chicken)
*pork sausage
*pork spareribs

DAIRY
hard cheeses

Carbohydrates

VEGGIES
carrots
corn
peas
potato (baked, mashed, or boiled)
pumpkin
rutabaga
turnips
winter squash

FRUITS
applesauce
apricot
banana
cantaloupe
cranberries
figs
fruit cocktail
guava
kumquat
mango
papaya
pineapple
prunes
raisins
watermelon

DIET TEAS OR SODA—BEWARE!!!

There is no question that sugar substitutes such as Nutrasweet call for a small amount of insulin. These products, marketed to the low-fat, diet-obsessed crowd, have the same deleterious effect as sugar in the raw. Keeping the need for sweets going, a quick sip of that diet drink gives your tongue that sweet sensation, and your body responds immediately as if sugar/carb were on the way, triggering a small release of insulin. A client of mine suspected this effect when she stopped drinking diet fruit-flavored iced tea for a week. The result? She lost five pounds immediately. This tendency to put on puffy weight is the calling card of her Metabolic Mix-Up, the same mechanism that's behind her stubborn high cholesterol and blood pressure and can lead her to the diabetic door if she's not careful.

STARCHY CARBS, LEGUMES AND GRAINS

bagels
cereals
  bran flakes
  Grainfield cereals
  Grape-Nuts
  puffed rice
  puffed wheat
  raisin bran
  shredded wheat
  sugared cereals
  Total
  Wheat Chex
  Wheaties
corn bread
crackers (white flour)
English muffins

pasta
refried beans
waffles
white flour breads

Condiments

French, Russian, blue cheese, green goddess dressings
half-and-half
heavy cream
honey mustard
ketchup
nondairy creamer
sugar

Beverages

alcoholic beverages
beer
Crystal Light
soda (including diet sodas containing maltodextrins and dex-
    trose)
diet tea drinks
wine

IT JUST MAKES SENSE

Just take the first step, and begin with Basic Balance. You will
become accustomed to eating the right foods frequently,
throughout the day. As you become exposed to the power of the
foods, you will feel stronger and happier. Even though we are
intimately familiar with food—involved in it and surrounded by
it—we often lose sight of how the foods we eat set the stage for
our daily performance. Yet when I use the analogy of money to
underscore the power of food, my clients always understand—

everybody relates to money. I'd like you to consider this figure: $15,500. What does it say? Right—$15,500. Now I am just going to make one little change and move the decimal point two places to the left: $155. Which would you rather have—$15,500 or $155? Of course, you are no fool! See the huge impact a small movement can have? By simply moving the decimal two *little* places the value of the figure was altered enormously. Well, it is not very different with your foods. Your food is your decimal point.

The simple mistake of eating a peach in the morning instead of an apple will create ripples all day long. And for some of us it becomes a tidal wave, in which our cravings and emotional ups and downs can drown us. Food is a science and until we understand it as such we remain at the mercy of those not-so-innocent raisins in our hot oatmeal breakfast. I know that Mother told you it was good for you, healthy fuel for a day's work, but she was only repeating what *her* mother told *her*. Time to join the twenty-first century and let the power of food and all its secrets be revealed to you and those you love. For some of you Basic Balance may take two weeks; for others, it may take only three or four days. Be patient, be kind—to yourself, that is. Everyone's chemistry is different and trust you will know when you are in Basic Balance! In the next chapter you will go to the next level—*your better balance*—where carbohydrates will no longer control your life.

CHAPTER 6

Step Two: Becoming Carb-Careful

NOT ONE MORE THING

Carb-Careful is not just about lowering blood pressure or cholesterol or reducing your risk of type 2 diabetes, it's about living and loving. Denise initially came to see me because she "didn't want to feel sick anymore." Although she was only moderately overweight at 149 pounds and 5 feet 4 inches, she had the classic signs of the Metabolic Mix-Up: She wanted to lose weight but couldn't; her extra pounds were wrapped around her middle, creating the typical apple shape; and her cholesterol would not go down, even though she ate a heart-healthy diet. She'd been doing Basic Balance, but it was clear to me that she needed to do more to lock her blood sugar into place. Despite her high-fiber, low-fat diet, her cholesterol levels were still too high, and she was still vulnerable to starches and sweets.

When I suggested that she might be ready to get Carb-Careful, at first she resisted. "I no longer feel like I am living in someone else's body, but I am not sure that I can give up one more thing!" I could hear the frustration in her voice and understood that it was her insulin resistance talking. She was not yet in better balance and was still being controlled by her chemistry. Trying to reassure her, I asked her why she *should* take the next step, suggesting that she was just fine where she was. After contemplating my question for a moment, she reconsidered and said, "I am feeling better since starting Basic Balance, but most of all I really don't want to be sick. I would like to lower my blood pressure and cholesterol—and I especially hate the way I look."

Denise not only answered my question, she answered her own. Her health had already begun to improve with Basic Balance, but she believed she could feel even better. I wanted her to reach that place where her blood sugar balance was so reliable, that she was finally free to live her life. She just needed to take the next step and become Carb-Careful.

STEP UP TO CARB-CAREFUL

You may be wondering why you need Carb-Careful if you've already stabilized your blood sugar in Basic Balance. It's a good question. Essentially, for those of us with the mix-up, we need to pay even more attention to the triggers that might upset the Basic Balance. Carb-Careful assures that we lock our Basic Balance into place so that we finally cut the cord from our damaging chemistry. Once we are in Carb-Careful, we are truly controlling our chemistry and are no longer swept up on the flying carbohydrate carpet.

As you know, balancing your blood sugar helps to dramatically reduce your carbohydrate cravings. For those of you who may not yet have developed overt medical or visual symptoms (remember the apple shape?) that signal insulin resistance, Basic Balance may be enough to achieve blood sugar control, eliminate most carb cravings, and support your overall health. But for many of us with the Metabolic Mix-Up, we need to step up to Carb-Careful in order to quiet this chemical call once and for all. If you are like Denise, you may feel much, much better after Basic Balance, but you shouldn't stop at just okay when you can move to a higher level. Why stop at good when you can get to great?

Carb-Careful will:

• Lower your cholesterol
• Lower your blood pressure
• Increase your vitality throughout the day
• Give you more stamina without the peaks and valleys
• Define a better body composition
• Reduce the signs of biological aging
• Provide you comfort and ease
• Ensure a greater sense of calm and serenity daily
• Improve your patience and goodwill
• Give a boost to your I-can-do confidence
• Put a spring in your step and a smile on your face
• Offer you lasting joie de vivre

Now why settle for anything less?

Let's see if you're ready to step up to Carb-Careful. Can you see yourself in these questions:

1. Do you feel better after Basic Balance, but have a suspicion that you could feel even better?
2. Are you doing Basic Balance accurately, but still wish you could have a sweeter fruit in the morning or a bag of pretzels as a snack after lunch?
3. Do you need to have a diet tea or soda in the afternoon as a pick-me-up even before you have your afternoon fruit?
4. Do you still find yourself not understanding why you can't just have a flavored yogurt for breakfast?
5. Does anyone have late-onset diabetes in your family?
6. Have you had a problem maintaining the weight you've lost in the last few years even though you haven't changed your diet or decreased your exercise?
7. Has the gap between your waist and your hips become smaller?
8. Do you have high cholesterol even though you eat a low-cholesterol diet?

9. Has your blood pressure recently begun to rise skyward?
10. Do you still get that puffy, bloated feeling after eating bread?
11. Can you never imagine putting your cereal and bananas back on the shelf indefinitely?

If you answered yes to even one of the eleven questions above, you are going to love how you feel when you become Carb-Careful. Just think: An even *better balance,* and all that goes with it, is within your reach. You are steps away from feeling so much happier in your life because of your improved health.

There are so many stories to share with you, it is sometimes hard to know which to choose. Different stories, different stars, but they all have in common a life-changing event: All the men and women who decided to become Carb-Careful have successfully conducted their chemistry to play a different tune. When Sam stepped up to Carb-Careful, he was amazed at the changes. Like so many of us, he kept struggling to feel better and could not really imagine how he was going to feel until he actually controlled his chemistry. As an accomplished violinist, he'd always been a driven man, demanding tremendous energy and results from himself. And this determination has paid off: He is very successful, receiving much acclaim from his peers in the highly competitive world of classical music. But as a self-proclaimed control freak, the only thing in his life Sam couldn't seem to control was his eating habits.

When he first came to see me he was about forty-five pounds overweight, and though he is only in his early forties, he had developed high cholesterol and high blood pressure, causing his physician to warn him that his family history put him at risk. And that's how he arrived on my doorstep—a high-risk package.

After two and a half months of working together and doing Basic Balance, he had lost twenty-five of those original forty-five pounds. He was happy with this, but in the coming months, losing the other twenty pounds became a struggle. Frustrated and disappointed, he kept complaining to me, asking me why he hadn't lost all the weight he desired.

It seemed that his chemistry was holding Sam back: I suspected that he had not fallen far from his family tree and that though he had achieved many positive results from Basic Balance, he could not maintain balanced blood sugar with just Step One. Having his blood pressure and cholesterol measured gave him more incentive to move into Carb-Careful. While his numbers were lower since he'd begun to follow Basic Balance, they had not yet improved to the point where he could come off his medications. His profile, typical of the mix-up, pointed to the distinct possibility that we would have to roll back the carbs further. Once these trigger foods were reduced, he would not mind—in fact he would feel so much better. If this were indeed the right level for him, he would not miss them very much at all and he would probably be free of his need for medications.

Sam's story depicts the typical person who needs to step up to Carb-Careful. With Basic Balance he improved his blood sugar balance, lost some weight, and felt better than he had in the past. But something was still not right. He wanted to achieve more—remember that driven personality? Where were the huge rewards that I had promised him? Sure he had lost some weight, but not all. Yes, he did feel better, but not great. After four days of Carb-Careful, he could barely wait to ask, "Will this incredible feeling last?" Yes. The answer is yes. This is no mistake; it's not an accident. You are becoming *better balanced,* and you are making this happen by redirecting your chemistry.

After just a week, Sam walked into my office and said, "I feel so different somehow—cleaner, lighter, and so less interested in all the food around me! I finally get it!" What Sam had finally understood was that food had remained powerful beyond his imagination because he had still been igniting his Metabolic Mix-Up. He realized that in order to feel really good, in order to get all his numbers in balance, he had to take another step: He had to become Carb-Careful.

By becoming Carb-Careful, you will calm down your chemistry to such a degree that you will no longer be prey to the insulin insult that has been hemming in your energy level and cutting yourself off from your full potential. You will not only feel the surge of energy that you first experienced in Basic Balance, you will realize you can rely on this feeling each and every day. Once you have moved away from the foods that have triggered your Metabolic Mix-Up, you will experience a dramatic improvement in your health and no task will seem beyond you, no country too big for you to roam.

IT'S RISKY BUSINESS TO STOP SHORT

Skipping the Carb-Careful step will backfire for those of us with the Metabolic Mix-Up. Rest assured, if your metabolic condition is not controlled, then illness almost surely will follow. Your heightened cholesterol, high blood pressure, exhaustion, and overweight may be signals from your Metabolic Mix-Up that serious illness is on the way. By working the steps of the Midlife Miracle Diet, you just may avoid such life-threatening diseases as type 2 diabetes, stroke, heart disease, and cancer.

BECOMING CARB-CAREFUL

Now is the time to go the distance and lock into place that good chemistry once and for all. However, this second step should only be taken if you're *already* in Basic Balance, which usually takes between three and five days. If you try to become Carb-Careful without taking this step, you will still be wildly craving carbs, and as a result, you will be unhappy, miserable, and furious with me for telling you to do this and furious with yourself for even trying.

The instructions for becoming Carb-Careful are similar to those of Basic Balance, so some of the breakfast, lunch, and dinner choices will seem familiar. However, there are crucial changes built into Carb-Careful around the need to roll back carbs in your day. Pay attention to the specifics of each meal; the actual changes are highlighted in your Remove These and Add These lists below. Use these lists as a guide to choose foods, but, of course, consult your Giant Food List for more choices. The main thrust of becoming Carb-Careful is to roll back the carbs, so most of the directions are designed to help accomplish this task.

Remove These

Bread and cereal out of breakfast
Fruit out of morning, if you can

Add These

Veggies to breakfast
Protein to breakfast
Partner remaining fruit snacks with protein

If you don't change what you are doing, you can't change what you are feeling. You have to talk to your chemistry. Becoming Carb-Careful takes work, but not more work than it's worth. And remember that the same thing that can drive you crazy because your weight won't behave can also lead to type 2 diabetes and premature aging.

And know that once you have reached *better balance* (the goal of Carb-Careful) you can then reintroduce some of your favorite carbohydrates, as long as you are accompanying them with pure-power veggies and protein. But first you need to lock in your state of good blood sugar and let your body know this balance, really know it, in a way you can rely on. Some of you may continue to be sensitive to carbs. If this is the case, know that the Supplement Solution in the next chapter will help lock balance in place.

Remember, the meals suggested below are samples. You will find more recommendations for menu ideas at the end of this chapter and, of course, your Giant Food List contains a complete list of inspiring food choices. Be creative!

THE DYNAMIC DUO

To make sure that you are working the steps in the best possible way, remember to do two things:

1. Drink plenty of water
2. Keep writing in your journal.

Breakfast

How to Eat

- **Remove starchy carbs at breakfast.** The first instruction for breakfast is to roll back carbs by taking the cereal and bread out of breakfast. You will be surprised to find that you don't miss these highly reactive starchy carbohydrates and all you'll feel is less needy and more in control.
- **Add veggies to breakfast.** Veggies supply you with a controlled release of sugar. Their high-fiber content helps your body to use the energy from these carbohydrates without shooting you into the outer stratosphere. You need this important lift to help you start your day. It's not necessary to rely on your usual Hard Chew; choose something more interesting, more fun from your pure-power list.
- **Continue to include protein.** The proteins will give you a quality start to your day.

What to Eat
Egg-white omelet made with mushrooms, broccoli, onion, and melted soy cheddar cheese

Chicken, fish, or your favorite pure-power protein
Low-fat cottage cheese, cherry tomatoes and slices of cucumber

Morning Snacks

How to Eat

- **Hard Chew veggies are stand-alone snacks.** These veggies will always be your better midmorning snack choice. Choose one or two from your pure-power list.
- **Partner your fruit.** If you are keeping fruit as a morning Hard Chew snack, then you need to add a high quality, low-fat protein to slow down the call for insulin that the sugar in the fruit ignites.

What to Eat

Any Hard Chew veggie (Go for them in the raw: fennel bulbs, celery, or string beans.)
Apple with a dollop of unsweetened nut butter (peanut or almond)
Pear with a generous spoonful of low-fat cottage cheese or
Slice of turkey

VEGGIES AND FRUITS ARE CARBS

You can enjoy fruits and vegetables if you a) choose fruits that are lower in glucose (less reactive); b) choose veggies and fruits that are high in fiber.

Lunch

How to Eat

- **Remove starchy carbs at lunch.** Since you are still vulnerable this early in the day to triggering too much insulin release, leaving you to deal with your reactions for the rest of the day, you should keep rolling back your carbs instead. This means no bread, rice, or potatoes at lunch. These are among the most seductive temptations. By avoiding them altogether, you lock in your Better Balance.

- **Include protein and veggies.** Put together a plate with a reasonable portion of protein and lots of low-starch, high-fiber veggies.
- **Add a salad.** A salad made of crudités—red or green peppers, radishes, celery, string beans, and broccoli dressed with a reasonable amount of salad dressing made of olive oil, vinegar, and your favorite herbs—is a wonderful way to include even more low-starch veggies without incurring the wrath of your mix-up.

What to Eat

Turkey wrapped around asparagus spears with red roasted pepper on top

Tuna made with vinegar, Dijon mustard, and dill (or any favorite herbs)

Tofu masked with a little bit of oil to make creamy soy sauce, garlic, and chopped veggies

Soy burger topped with melted soy cheese and a slice of tomato

Always add a salad or some other leafy green dish.

FRENCH WISDOM

The French eat a salad with oil and vinegar with most meals. Just another healthy habit since vinegar greatly reduces the reactive potential of the rest of the meal.

Afternoon Snacks

How to Eat

- **Stand-alone veggies.** Can't you tell that I'm absolutely smitten with veggies? They pack a pure-power punch without leaving you vulnerable. What could be better on your way to Better Balance?
- **Partner fruit with protein.** Fruit can be either Hard or Soft Chew, but you must combine it with a protein to continue to lock in your balanced blood sugar. Try an apple with some almonds or berries with some yogurt. Check your Giant Food List for other great ideas.
- **Late dinners require a second snack.** If you know in advance that you will be eating dinner later than 8:00 P.M., you risk upsetting your blood sugar balance unless you have a second afternoon snack. Of course, veggies are the best choice, adding a small amount of protein at this late hour.

What to Eat

broccoli spears dipped in low-fat yogurt, seasoned with mustard or dill
cucumber chunks
blueberries with a dollop of low-fat cottage cheese
peach slices with a slice of soy cheese

THE ELECTRIC FORCE OF FIBER

We know that fiber helps to keep the digestive tract on track, but did you know that it also slows the metabolism of carbohydrates, which in turn slows down the call for insulin? The more fiber in the carbohydrate, the better it is for those of us with the Metabolic Mix-Up.

> ### BE CREATIVE AND HAVE FUN
>
> You have a wide variety of foods and condiments available to you. Use them! Don't be afraid to be inventive. Get familiar with your Giant Food List and browse through the cookbooks (see page 189–90). And remember, these foods are just the beginning.

Dinner

How to Eat

• **Dinner is made up of protein and veggies.** Look at your plate: Is it mostly high-quality protein and veggies?

• **Include a complex carbohydrate at dinner every two or three nights if you wish.** By continuing to limit your starchy carbs, spacing out their frequency, and choosing wisely, you can test how much they may trigger your Metabolic Mix-Up.

• **If you're still feeling reactive to carbs,** and haven't quite locked in your Better Balance, be prepared to skip the starchy carb at dinner a little while longer. You'll know when you can have those red bliss potatoes or lentil pilaf, and it's worth waiting for.

What to Eat

Grilled chicken breast on a bed of braised radicchio with
 steamed zucchini, yellow summer squash, and onions sprinkled with olive oil, basil, and oregano

Sauteed spinach and cauliflower with shrimp or scallops,
 adding garlic for flavor

Broiled flounder with a side of Swiss chard and broccolini and
 a salad of endive and arugula with mustard vinaigrette

Steamed shrimp and Chinese vegetables (bok choy, water
 chestnuts, broccoli, mushrooms)

As you move from Basic Balance to Carb-Careful, bear in mind that you may respond less or more quickly, depending on your personal profile. It may take some of you two weeks to get into Basic Balance (Step One); while for others, it may take only three or four days. The same holds true for how long it may take you to become Carb-Careful (Step Two). For some of you, it may take one week; for others it may take three or four. This does not mean that quicker is better or that you are more or less successful. The length of time it takes you to reach *better balance* is merely a reflection of how reactive your body chemistry is. It's difficult to predict the impact of your unique body chemistry and how it interplays with your personality, drive, and other things going on in your life and the world around you. But I do know this for certain: You will become convinced when you pay attention to how your body responds to certain foods, enabling you to predict your future reactions.

By becoming Carb-Careful, you will feel much less connected to the foods, experiencing a new level of health that goes beyond feeling good. As you continue to roll back your carbs, and lock your *better balance* into place, you are moments away from a state of enduring harmony that is your goal. And remember, while there is no one timetable, there is one outcome: You are the ultimate captain of your body's ship. So keep your eyes on the vast, wondrous sea ahead of you, and know that your goal should be the sweet harmony that becoming Carb-Careful can bring. With the help of the Supplement Solution in step 3, you can be even more assured of smooth sailing ahead.

TAKE AN INTERMISSION: HOW ARE YOU DOING?

Take some time now to see how close you are to *better balance*. Respond to the questions below and see how you are doing.

1. Have your blood pressure and LDL decreased?
2. Are you no longer tired in the afternoon or after dinner?
3. Do you get up in the morning with a smile on your face, excited to greet the day?

4. Do you find yourself spending less time and energy sweating the small stuff?
5. Are you newly interested in tucking in your shirts or dressing that trimmer waist in a new belt?
6. Have you lost weight around your middle or kept off what you lost in *Basic Balance?*
7. Are you no longer looking for foods, never mind longing for them?

If you answered even one question with a yes, then you are approaching *better balance.*

LET THE NEGOTIATIONS BEGIN

Once you are in better balance, you have the power to negotiate with your chemistry to reintroduce some of the carbs that you had to roll back. With your blood sugar stable, you should be less vulnerable to those powerhouse triggers. You should also be more comfortable about using the information properly to slow down your reactions.

Use the following suggestions as guidelines:

1. Look at your Giant Food List and choose carbs that are less reactive and fall in the pure-power or middle-road groups.
2. Introduce the foods one by one, starting slowly, so that you can see just how reactive you may be.
3. Make sure that this carb is escorted through the meal by pure-power veggies and protein.
4. Stay with this level of carbs for a week or two to see how you feel before reintroducing potentially more reactive food.
5. Then if you wish, select a carb that's slightly more reactive from your middle-road foods on your Giant Food List. How do you feel? Are you still in balance?

6. **If weight loss is important to you, you may want to stick with those carbs in Pure Power or continue to roll back carbs as directed on Carb-Careful.**

The Carb-Careful Solution has built-in choices and a lot of flexibility, encouraging you to become adventurous. Once you step up to supplement synergy (Step Three) and exercise euphoria (Step Four) you will discover even more choices as you become even less reactive to carbohydrates.

CARB-CAREFUL CREDO

Never have a starchy or sweet carbohydrate without a protein. Whether you are eating lentils or potatoes, having that occasional good-for-the-soul glass of wine, or dessert; eating these carbs without partnered protein is like leaving a young child in a playground without supervision. Unguided, these carbs will make you run wild. If you indulge in a glass of wine, accompany it with some low-fat cheese. If you have beans or lentils with a meal, make sure you include some protein: a piece of fish, chicken—even beef—and vegetables, of course.

SAMPLE MEALS FOR CARB-CAREFUL

Here is another few days' worth of sample meals. Keep in mind the variations of time and how they impact your snacks and meals. The exact times are meant as suggestions; it's more important to focus on eating at regular intervals, which will ensure *better balance.* And remember: Snacks are not meals. Don't go overboard and eat too much—about one quarter the amount of a meal-size portion is adequate.

Day One

Breakfast: (7:30 A.M.)	Sliced turkey
	Soy cheese wrapped around peppers
Hard Chew snack: (9:30 A.M.)	Celery
Hard Chew snack: (11:00 A.M.)	Fennel chunks with low-fat cheese
Lunch: (12:30 P.M.)	Small pop-top can tuna, packed in spring water, with lettuce, tomato, radish, and dry-roasted peppers with vinaigrette dressing
Soft or Hard Chew snack: (3:30 P.M.)	Tangerine with raw almonds
Dinner: (6:00 P.M.)	Chinese takeout: steamed vegetables, chicken, and brown rice

Day Two

Breakfast: (7:30 A.M.)	Scrambled egg whites and tofu with tomato salsa
Hard Chew snack: (9:30 A.M.)	Kirby cucumber with low-fat ricotta
Lunch: (12:30 P.M.)	Chinese chicken salad made with steamed or grilled chicken with water chestnuts and scallions in a sauce *without* sugar and with a few celery sticks.
Soft or Hard Chew snack: (3:30 P.M.)	Kirby cucumber

Dinner: (7:00 P.M.)   Baked blue fish in a lemon dill
marinade

Side of mushrooms and peppers

Salad with oil and vinegar

Blueberries for dessert

NOTE: *A small amount of high-quality protein may be added to veggie
snacks if desired. Be sure to add the protein when dinner is after 7:00 P.M.*

Day Three

Breakfast: (7:30 A.M.)   Mushroom and spinach omelet with
herbs de provence

Hard Chew snack: (9:30 A.M.)   Pear and slice of soy cheese

Lunch: (12:30 P.M.)   Steamed lobster

Salad with oil and vinegar

Steamed broccoli

Soft or Hard Chew: (3:30 P.M.)   Green beans

Dinner: (6:00 P.M.)   Baked Cornish hen, skinless

Lentil pilaf with wheat berries and
almonds

Brussels sprouts, blanched and then
sauteed in oil and garlic

Small mixed green salad with endive

Day Four

Breakfast: (6:00 A.M.)   Rye bread with low-fat cottage
cheese, sprinkled with dill and
topped with sliced tomato

Snack: (8:00 A.M.)	Pear and almonds
Snack: (10:00 A.M.)	Handful from Hard Chew grab bag
Lunch: (12:30 P.M.)	Green salad, red peppers, cucumbers with Italian dressing
	Shrimp salad with celery chunks
	Carrot sticks
Snack: (3:30 P.M.)	Strawberries and blueberries with dollop of plain yogurt
Dinner: (7:00 P.M.)	Grilled veal chop
	Sauteed green beans with dill
	Tossed green salad with sliced purple onion, dressed with olive oil, vinegar, garlic, and mustard

Day Five

Breakfast: (7:30 A.M.)	Melted low-fat mozzarella cheese on seven-grain bread
Snack: (10:00 A.M.)	Veggie grab bag
Lunch: (12:30 P.M.)	Caesar salad
	Grilled salmon steak
	Steamed brussels sprouts
	Kirby cucumber chunks
Snack: (3:30 P.M.)	Apple and blueberry fruit salad with dollop of low-fat plain yogurt
Dinner: (6:30 P.M.)	Asparagus vinaigrette
	Filet of sole with fines herbes
	Mashed butternut squash
	Steamed broccoli

BETTER BALANCE

My job is to get you into Carb-Careful. It's up to you to stay there. But as I've been saying all along, once you have the sweet taste of *better balance,* you're not going to need me to motivate you to continue working the steps. You will feel satisfied and sated. As Beth, a healthy middle-aged woman who climbed Mount Kilimanjaro over the summer, reported after rolling back her carbs, "I feel different, somehow uplifted. It's not just from climbing the heights." She then told me about having just had a wonderful lunch at the City Bakery Café, describing in great detail the fresh ingredients and exciting taste of the food. "You know," she went on to explain, "there were incredible cakes and breads on the bakery side of the café and most incredible of all was a huge mountain of cookie dough in the center of the room. I mean huge—really huge! Remember how I used to bake for friends just so I could eat some dough? Well there it was—a looming mound of my favorite indulgence—and I was looking, but I wasn't longing!" That's the promise of becoming Carb-Careful: no more cravings—only energy—as your body builds healthy reserves and prepares you for a future of vibrant health.

CHAPTER 7

Step Three: The Supplement Solution

SPECIAL NOTE

If you are currently taking medication, consult your physician before taking any supplements.

LET SUPPLEMENTS SERENADE YOU

Not too long ago, I celebrated a special occasion with my husband and friends at Picholine, my favorite New York City restaurant. The pretty surroundings, incredible food, and good company were ingredients enough to stimulate the food sensualist in me. I was not there to eat just salad and plain grilled fish. I was there to enjoy myself. In other words, this was not a place to go on a restrictive diet.

And I did not come undressed. Just as I had pulled out my favorite outfit in preparation for the evening, I also had talked to my chemistry. I was in very balanced blood sugar but still ready for some food fun. In the preceding weeks, I had been researching and reviewing the most recent literature on supplements. In response to this latest information, I changed the combinations of my supplements and their amounts. When the night for the special dinner arrived, I was excited to see if I could ease the food life of a classic Metabolic Mix-Up person like me.

I ordered a delicious meal: tournedos of salmon with horseradish, cucumbers, and salmon caviar along with a salad of organic green-market lettuces, dressed with a Banyols-shallot vinaigrette and garden herb dressing. And although I managed to pass up their delectable breads, I did have dessert—their famous Warm Michele Chocolate Tart. Normally, I would pay dearly for such a meal: In twenty-four hours I would have gained two or three pounds, become bloated, outgrown the smaller hole on my belt, and felt terrible. But the next day, I hadn't gained a single pound and felt better than ever for a morning after—not as well as when I don't indulge, but still reasonably well. I was feeling grateful that the supplements had done their job to escort the insulin with its glucose package into the cell. Just as the research had reported, I had clearly had a gentler reaction to these trigger foods.

The morning after, and throughout the next day, I felt an energy that was lower than my usual high level (a normal reaction to eating trigger carbs such as the wine and dessert), but I felt so much better than I normally would have. No mountains had moved and my blood sugar foundation was not cracking. What a wonderful feeling!

This is just the beginning of the story of the supplement solution that has been waiting to be written. We now have access to a much greater understanding of how supplements can interact with and help control insulin resistance. Recent ongoing research has shown that we can alter and improve the body's mechanism to utilize insulin at the cellular site and also to help achieve a body composition that looks, feels, and *is* healthy. As you saw in Chapter Four, weight numbers do not necessarily tell the whole story. You will contribute more to your overall health if you increase your lean muscle mass and decrease your fat than if you simply lose weight. The more muscle and the less fat you have, the more effective your metabolism and the more your insulin resistance is kept in check. As you will see, supplements are one of the key ingredients that help you improve the ratio of your body fat to lean muscle mass, allowing you to better your body composition. And if that were not enough, an improvement in body composition helps to reduce your biological age so you not only look and feel younger than your chronological age, but you also reduce the risk of age-related diseases.

But I would be remiss if I didn't point out that there are inherent dangers to supplements, too. In the past few years there has been a lot written and discussed about supplements. Such supplements as alpha lipoic acid and chromium are being bandied about as quick fixes that ensure permanent weight loss and fat reduction. And while I think this is a good sign that people are recognizing and becoming more open to the idea of supplements, I also worry that these compounds are being used as silver bullets—a one-pill-cures-all approach to losing weight and optimizing health. I feel very strongly that you need to know not only what these supplements can do for you but also how to use them in the best possible way.

Though we all share the menacing Metabolic Mix-Up, we still remain individuals with unique biochemistry formed by individual family histories, lifestyle, exercise, and eating habits. We all respond to stress differently—both internal stresses and those of the environment. You can look back at your profile quiz in Chapter Three to evaluate your own degree of the Metabolic Mix-Up.

I have a personal interest in this subject for myself as well as for all of you who share this disorder of metabolism. Without a doubt, supplements will impact how you feel. I designed this part of the program considering all of the most up-to-date information regarding the long-term health benefits of using supplements. And if you've been feeling better doing Basic Balance and Carb-Careful, just ready yourself for changing your destiny to one of superior health, growing energy, and lifelong well-being. You won't need a crystal ball to believe that you can shape your future.

The Supplement Solution gets at the very heart of your Metabolic Mix-Up by helping to redesign your chemistry. It both redirects the signal at the cell door to let in the insulin and facilitates the transport of glucose throughout the cell. Four very important supplements are the main engineers of this chemical reworking. I call them the four-star medley.

The four-star medley is followed by my A-list of supplements that I recommend for everyone. This basic grouping of vitamins and minerals work behind the scenes to control your chemistry even more effectively.

The Supplement Solution can be tailored to your specific needs. Although we all share the Metabolic Mix-Up, there is no universal guide to dosage or frequency of supplements that will cover all people's needs or take into consideration their particular combination of factors. The amount, frequency, and combination of supplements that work best for you are based on you: your history, your lifestyle, your reaction to stress. You have a general guide on what supplements to take and when to take them, based on many clients' responses. You can follow the directions to individualize a program that suits you specifically. For instance, if you exercise less than three times a week, you may want to increase your dosage of CLA and alpha lipoic acid. Or if you, like me, enjoy indulging your food sensualist every now and then at a special occasion, then you may need to increase your dosages of chromium and vanadyl sulfate, making sure they are squarely in place to help you lessen the impact of the delicious event. Embracing the Supplement Solution allows you to move through life with flexibility, versatility, and a freedom from the restrictive, limiting diet programs of the past. The supplements have the power to allow you to open all doors so the world becomes your own precious oyster.

FOODS ARE NOT ENOUGH

It is not possible to obtain all the nutrients you need to support a vibrant, healthy body. You need supplements. Just look at what supplements can do for you:

- Aid in proper digestion
- Improve metabolism
- Supply essential vitamins and nutrients that are depleted in food sources

- Reverse loss of nutrients caused by handling of foods, including storage and cooking
- Supply nutrients without additional calories
- Offset a somewhat sedentary lifestyle
- Overcome genetic predisposition for overweight, high blood pressure, and high cholesterol
- Mitigate the effects of a toxic environment
- Lessen the impact of stress on our bodies
- Enhance body composition

HOW SUPPLEMENTS WORK

The first two steps of the Midlife Miracle Diet focused on reshaping your eating habits by redesigning when you eat and how you eat, especially by curbing and partnering your intake of carbohydrates. The first two steps make sure you are in balanced blood sugar. Without that, nothing else can happen. Step Three, the Supplement Solution, builds on your state of good blood sugar and enhances the program's impact on your metabolic system.

Supplements can tame your Metabolic Mix-Up in five essential ways:

1. They can open the cell's doors to allow in the necessary insulin with its glucose cargo.
2. Supplements help the cells take up glucose by facilitating the glucose transport and distribution throughout the cells.
3. Supplements help you burn fat more efficiently, which increases your lean muscle mass and enhances your body composition. Together, these effects help decrease insulin resistance.
4. They aid in the metabolism and breakdown of carbohydrates.
5. Supplements protect against free radicals, the dangerous positive ions that attach themselves to fat, protein, and other molecules in the body and cause not only oxidative stress related to accelerated aging but also some forms of cancer.

I'm not asking you to memorize these functions, but it is important to know that supplements are working on the front lines of your chemistry, getting your body to function and behave as though the Metabolic Mix-Up were not a part of your history and the insulin insult not part of your destiny.

ARE YOU READY FOR THE SUPPLEMENT SOLUTION?

1. Do you pride yourself on never taking vitamins?
2. Do you let your children out of their one-a-day vitamins even though the pediatrician has recommended them?
3. Can you remember the last time you took your vitamins two days in a row?
4. Do you find you have no time to pack or room to put your vitamins when you're traveling or on vacation?
5. Do you believe that vitamins are an unnecessary expense because you get enough nutrients from the food you eat?

If you have answered yes to even one of these questions, you may have to remind yourself a few times that you really want to give supplements a try. If you answered yes to more than two, then you are probably still resistant. This was the case with Mark, who had been doing remarkably well as he worked the steps. When he first came in to see me he could barely walk upstairs without becoming completely exhausted and out of breath. His lack of vibrancy was a clear marker of his poor health. After six weeks, he was feeling dramatically stronger and had much more stamina. When he felt he'd reached *better balance*, he wanted to include more carbs in his diet, but he started to forget to take his vitamins and other supplements. He was planning his increase (in carbs), his decrease (in supplements), and his demise all in one breath.

Luckily, he caught himself before it was too late. Putting the supplements back into place, he was able to increase his complex carbohydrates without increasing his risk. He could be comfortable with the knowledge that he was doing everything possible to maintain vibrant health by continuing to reorganize his foods, lose weight, and increase his exercise. Remember, proper foods, vitamins, and exercise work synergistically.

THE FOUR-STAR MEDLEY: GETTING TO THE CORE OF YOUR METABOLIC MIX-UP

There are four major supplements that are instrumental in the reduction of insulin resistance and hyperinsulinemia. These four supplements, when properly used, will let you eat reasonable amounts of carbohydrates without paying so high a price. As your cells begin to let in the insulin that had been blocked, you will begin to feel changes in your body, so please pay close attention to how you feel. You should feel more at ease, but if instead you become edgy or irritable (a sign that your blood sugar may have dropped too low) or if you still feel lethargic and tired, then you may need to adjust the amount of the supplement accordingly. The appropriate dosages vary depending on the carbohydrate content in your meals and the amount of exercise you are averaging. As you begin the four-star medley, use the charts starting on page 132 as guides for the appropriate dosage for you.

1. Alpha Lipoic Acid. This supplement is instrumental in the proper processing of carbohydrates, making your cells more efficient in the uptake of glucose and resetting the transport signal so the cell responds to insulin. Also, recent research suggests that alpha lipoic acid will lower blood pressure by increasing the activity of calcium.

2. CLA (Conjugated Linoleic Acid): CLA activates two different receptor sites on a cell nucleus that play an important role in allowing the glucose in. In this way, CLA has the ability both to decrease body fat significantly and increase lean muscle mass (it's a fat burner). Also, when taken with alpha lipoic acid, CLA raises the vesicles of the cell to the surface so the cell is better able to receive and distribute the glucose. Together these functions help diminish your insulin resistance. Recently, a U.S. patent recognized CLA as an official fat burner that worked without exercise.

3. Chromium Polynicotinate: Chromium is rarely abundant in the typical American diet and sugar actually diminishes whatever amount we may have. It is necessary to facilitate the metabolism of fat (remember, it's also a fat burner), enabling the insulin to bind to the appropriate cell receptors so glucose can enter cells.

4. Vanadyl Sulfate: This supplement, instrumental in opening the cellular switch, works best in combination with chromium, manganese, and zinc (contained in your multivitamin) for most blood sugar problems, especially balancing low blood sugar, so be sure to take the rest of your vitamins.

Since you are not in my office, and I cannot adjust your vitamins to match your individual chemistry, it's up to you to stay aware of how you feel as you begin to slowly integrate supplements each day. But the thing you must remember most is to start slowly. Record your reactions to your foods in your journal, and at the end of a week, see if any patterns have developed. Again, rely on the charts that follow to guide you and make adjustments as needed. Always begin the supplement with the lower amount. More is not necessarily better. When Jill started the four-star medley, she used the lowest recommended amounts. In four and a half months she not only went from 159 to 139 pounds, but she also reduced her overall body fat from 27 percent to 18.9 percent, an exciting change for anyone. "I feel wonderful," she remarked. You too may feel wonderful as you enhance your body composition and increase your overall health, even with minimal amounts of supplements.

HOW YOU'RE EATING WILL DETERMINE YOUR NEED FOR CHROMIUM AND VANADYL SULFATE

Food combinations will affect your need for chromium and vanadyl sulfate. Follow these guidelines that give you specific instructions for how to adjust your supplements as needed.

- If you eat a meal of unrefined carbs (green, red, and yellow vegetables) with a reasonable portion of protein and complex carbs:

  Take once a day
      200 mcg of chromium
      2.5–5 mg of vandayl sulfate (vanadium)

- If you eat a mixed meal of high quality protein and veggies and a small amount of starchy carbs, and you are reacting to the carbs:

  Take twice a day
      200 mcg of chromium
      2.5–5 mg of vandayl sulfate (vanadium)

- If you eat a mixed meal of low- or midquality protein, starchy carbs, and few veggies, and your BMI is above 26 or your hip to waist ratio is 1:1 or higher:

  Take three times a day
      200 mcg of chromium
      2.5–5 mg of vandayl sulfate (vanadium)

IMPACT OF EXERCISE WILL AFFECT YOUR USE OF CLA AND ALPHA LIPOIC ACID

- If you exercise strenuously—working out 5 or more days a week:

  Skip
      CLA
      alpha lipoic acid

- If you exercise moderately—working out 3 days a week:

  Take once a day
      500 mg of CLA
      100 mg of alpha lipoic acid

- If you exercise minimally—working out 1 day a week:

  Take twice a day
  500 mg of CLA
  100 mg of alpha lipoic acid

- If you don't exercise at all:

  Take three times a day
  500 mg of CLA
  100 mg of alpha lipoic acid

THE INTERPLAY OF SUPPLEMENTS: WHERE DO YOU FIT IN?

Use the regular dosage amounts daily to guide your Supplement Solution. As you walk the steps and continue to monitor your reactions to foods and to exercise, and to use your supplements, you will see improvements in your all-around health. Don't take this as a sign to stop taking your supplements. Remember the synergy of the Carb-Careful Solution. The whole is greater than the sum of the parts. If you stop taking your supplements, you will hinder the synergy and hinder your health.

However, depending on *how* intensely you are working the steps, your amounts of supplements may vary according to these four factors:

- How reactive you are still feeling as you walk the steps
- The amount of carbohydrates you eat regularly
- If you indulge in a trigger food
- How often you exercise

THE A LIST: WHAT EVERYONE SHOULD TAKE

I make no bones about it: Almost everyone should take supplements. As you can see from the list of benefits above, the power of

---

UP THE VANADYL SULFATE WHEN YOU UP YOUR CARBS

If you're taking vanadyl sulfate only once a day, then be sure to take it with any meal that contains bread, pasta, rice, potatoes, or corn. You know, all those starchy little devils that make your blood sugar soar. It can also help to lessen the negative effects of the sugar in any dessert.

---

supplements is too strong to ignore. They don't just give you freedom to expand your eating repertoire, but they also reduce the chances of triggering the inevitable consequences of your Metabolic Mix-Up.

Unlike the four-star medley described above, my A-list includes the general supplements that everyone should take daily (all specified amounts are daily unless otherwise indicated). They include a good basic multivitamin, essential fatty acids (EFAs), magnesium, L-arginine, fat burners, and antioxidants. Together these supplements will synergize the way you eat, maximizing the effects of your change in diet and enhancing your overall health.

1. Multivitamin

All multivitamins are not alike, so be sure you check the label. And while there is some variation in the amounts of the different formulas, don't be concerned if my recommended amounts differ somewhat from yours. This is just a sample of the many acceptable formulas that are available. You can always add to your multi or change brands next month. My A-list multivitamin is just a sample of the many acceptable formulas that are available. A simple basic multivitamin could look like this:

Vitamin	Amount
A (as beta-carotene)	10,000 IU
D	400 IU
E	100 IU

Vitamin	Amount
K	60 mcg
C	150 mg
folic acid	400 mcg
B_1	1.5 mg
B_2	2 mg
B_3	2 mg
B_6	2 mg
B_{12}	100 mcg
pantothenic acid	50 mg
biotin	200 mcg

Mineral	Amount
calcium	25 mg
phosphorus	109 mg
iodine	150 mcg
*iron	10 mg
magnesium	7.2 mg
copper	3 mg
zinc	12 mg
manganese	500 mcg
potassium	40 mg
inositol	25 mg
chromium	100 mcg
molybdenum	25 mcg
selenium	100 mcg
boron	150 mcg

*NOTE: Postmenopausal women and mature men should not take any extra iron.

2. Essential fatty acids (EFAs) 2,000–4,000 mg
Essential fatty acids are critical for the health of your skin and hair, which is important to everyone, but they go beyond that.

Bs IN YOUR BONNET

All your B vitamins are important for the metabolism of carbs. Since they work together synergistically, it is usually a good idea to take them together in a single high-potency supplement. The main B vitamins in this group are B_1, B_2, B_3, B_6, B_{12}, biotin, pantothenic acid, folic acid, and choline. Check the label of your multivitamin; if you're not getting enough in the multi, take an additional 50 mg of B complex.

RDA: RIDICULOUS DAILY AMOUNTS

The RDA is the government's recommendation for a sufficient amount of a daily supplement. However, it often ignores biochemical individuality and environmental factors. Recent research suggest that the RDA figures are often insufficient and based on outdated information.

EFAs should be on your front line in the battle against your Metabolic Mix-Up. They help reduce blood pressure and raise the HDL (good cholesterol) while lowering the LDL (bad cholesterol). There are several types of essential fatty acids that may be part of your supplement, including omega-3 oils, especially fish oils and flaxseed oil. If the fish oil causes mild stomach distress, store the capsules in the freezer. They lose their fishy taste and won't make you burp. If you take a higher amount, then split the dosage during the day.

Warning: Essential Fatty Acids and Vitamin E Can Thin Blood
Do not take EFAs or vitamin E if you are taking blood thinners.

ESSENTIAL FATTY ACID FACTS

You can get some EFAs from foods: flaxseed (try grinding up flaxseeds as needed in a minigrinder for best results) and deepwater fish, such as salmon, sardines, and mackerel. Be sure to eat these foods two or three times a week; if not, then be sure to take your supplements.

---

3. Magnesium (magnesium glycinate) 100–200 mg
In addition to what may be found in your multi unless your multi already contains more than 100 mgs. With this form of magnesium, you should not experience any stomach or bowel upset. With other forms, you may have to reduce or split the dose.

4. L-arginine 1,000 mg
Two times daily. This supplement reduces fat tissue and helps to improve insulin sensitivity. It also stimulates the release of growth hormone and improves immune function.

5. Fat burners
This group of supplements is necessary not only to help with the reduction of fat but also to decrease insulin resistance. And anything that burns fat will eventually help to ease the entry or passage of the insulin into the cell. I suggest two main fat burners:

• **Acetyl L-carnitine or L-carnitine** 500–1,500 mg. An aminolike acid, this supplement metabolizes fat by helping to build skeletal muscle; it decreases dangerous triglycerides while increasing HDL (good cholesterol). It's also fuel for the heart by strengthening its muscle and reducing angina, or heart pain. Since it is so similar in structure to a protein, it's best to take L-carnitine away from proteins because amino acids compete for entry and absorption.

• **Inositol** 500 mg. Although grouped with the B vitamins, inositol is best taken on its own in order to ensure sufficient amount. This powerful supplement helps metabolize fat and transport it from the liver. It also helps maintain the circulatory system, reducing cholesterol levels and preventing hardening of the arteries. Another interesting feature of inositol is its ability to relieve depression and anxiety. However, if you have been diagnosed with bipolar disorder avoid this supplement.

STRESS STOMPER

Pantothenic acid, also known as B_5, fights the debilitating effects of stress by supporting your adrenal gland functions. Next time you hit a high-stress period—either on the job or at home—be sure to take your B vitamin group to replenish the pantothenic acid your body is using.

---

6. Antioxidants. These powerful supplements help protect against the free-radical damage that excess insulin can initiate. A free radical is an unstable, highly reactive molecule that is constantly looking for another molecule to bond with. When it literally steals an electron from its prey, that molecule is damaged. Antioxidants pair with these reactive molecules, preventing the damage free radicals can cause, including weakening your immune system and accelerating aging.

- **vitamin E**—400 IU. Check the amount in your multi; it may have levels that are lower than recommended.
- **vitamin C**—500–2,000 mg.
- **selenium**—100 mcg. Check your multi and do not exceed 200 mcg total. Levels beyond can be toxic.
- **grape seed or pycnogenol**—100–200 mg.

DAILY INSTRUCTIONS FOR YOUR SUPPLEMENT SOLUTION

Supplements are powerful so be sure you introduce them into your life with the utmost care. Here are my daily instructions:

• Introduce only one new supplement on any given day so that you can trace a possible reaction. If you're already taking a multivitamin and other supplements, continue their use, adding the new supplements one at a time. Check your multi to see if it includes additional amounts.

• Always begin with the lowest suggested dose, working your way slowly to a higher amount.

• Try to take supplements at the same time each day.

• You should take most vitamins with meals or directly after meals unless otherwise instructed on the label.

• Invest in vitamin cases in varying sizes so that you can bring your supplements with you wherever you go.

• Use small (3½ ounce) paper cups and place seven days' worth of supplements in 7 cups and store in the refrigerator. Line them up in two rows if you're taking vitamins twice a day.

Other considerations in purchasing supplements:

• Check the date on the supplement and make sure it has not expired.

• Purchase your supplements at a health food store or other market that you know has a regular turnover.

• Some reliable brands of vitamins include Metagenics, Twin Labs, and Country Life.

• Compare several brands and make sure you are getting the most for your money. Do not be seduced by lower prices. Quality is important and you may be getting what you pay for.

YOUR A LIST AT A GLANCE

Multivitamin
Essential fatty acids
Magnesium
L-arginine
Fat burners
Antioxidants

THE SYNERGY OF SUPPLEMENTS

Just like the whole of the Carb-Careful Solution, supplements are also synergistic: They work better in combination with one another, and their value increases tremendously in the company of the other steps. Since it is nearly impossible for foods to provide all the nutrients and ingredients for optimal metabolism and health, vitamins and minerals will enhance the effect of the program. We live in a challenging world in which supplements are an effective, important ingredient in helping you to build a natural environmental shield to protect your health and well-being. Why would you want to miss such an easy-to-catch brass ring? And you can embrace the supplement solution and pave your own way to magnificent health and a new-found joy in living. And there is more help ahead. You will see how exercise further enhances the effects of your supplement.

CHAPTER 8

Step Four: Exercise Euphoria

EXERCISE *IS* FOR EVERYONE

It never used to be like this. Exercisespeak used to go on only in the gym between jocks. Now, thanks to recent research and the media's power to spread the word, everyone is getting into the act—and just in the nick of time. The type 2 diabetes explosion this past decade is reason enough to pay attention to the power of exercise. The good news is that by including some type of workout routine in your life, one that increases fitness and muscle tone, you can reverse your insulin resistance, as well as decrease your hyperinsulinemia. Improving muscle tone can actually change the nature of your cells, helping to tame and control your Metabolic Mix-Up. And by taming your disruptive metabolism through exercise, you improve your overall health and offset accelerated aging. Plus, exercise will improve your body composition by increasing your lean muscle mass while decreasing your fat tissue. Now that you know the powerful potential of exercise, don't be surprised if that jump rope, pair of skates, or running shoes just leap out of the closet.

Exercise in any form—walking twenty to thirty minutes a day, swimming, participating in an endurance spin class—is a key element in making the program work at its optimum. The reason is

> ### IMPORTANT WARNING
>
> Everyone starting a new exercise program should check with his or her doctor before becoming much more physically active.

simple: By improving your body's ability to use insulin, you get to the very heart of your insulin resistance. And know this, too: By retraining your cells to welcome the insulin and its glucose passenger, you will experience the most amazing increase in your energy—and who wouldn't enjoy more of that?

For those of you who don't get excited by even *the idea* of a five-mile run or three sets of tennis, rock climbing, or an hour-long spin class, here's some more good news: You can be moderate. Recent research has proven that a mere brisk twenty-minute walk burns more fat calories than jogging or running. Why? Because the body prefers to use fat for fuel. Let the myth die here that you should carbo-load before working out. I know this news is going to disappoint the carb-craving masses who have embraced this myth as fact, but the only people who should consider carbo-loading are marathon runners or Olympic decathletes.

The benefits of reasonable, regular exercise don't stop there. There is even more good news: Studies show that low-intensity, prolonged exercise, such as a daily brisk walk of forty-five minutes to an hour, will substantially lower insulin levels and therefore reduce the risk of both diabetes and heart disease. With regular exercise, even after you've stopped working out, your body continues to burn calories more efficiently for hours afterward. Just think: After a few months of regular exercise, your body's metabolism will begin to burn calories at a higher rate *throughout* the day. And, of course, the more you exercise, the more muscle you build; and the more muscular you are, the more efficiently you will metabolize food and increase your energy.

The benefits of exercise go on and on. Exercise not only trims your body and gives you more energy, but it also has the power to elevate your mood. If you already exercise regularly (three to five times a week), then you are probably familiar with this effect: If you miss a day or two of workouts, your body not only begins to feel sluggish but you also feel more moody and less able to cope with the stresses of everyday life. But the euphoria of exercise comes from how you can reverse accelerated aging and improve the quality of your life by fighting against age-related diseases before they happen.

EXERCISE IS AN INTEGRAL PART OF THE MIDLIFE MIRACLE DIET. WHY? BECAUSE IT:

- Increases your metabolism
- Increases good cholesterol (HDL)
- Reduces insulin resistance
- Burns calories
- Slows osteoporosis
- Reduces stress
- Tones and strengthens muscles
- Helps you maintain steady weight loss
- Increases lung and heart capacity
- Gives you more joie de vivre

APPLE FIGURE NO MORE!

Basic Balance and Carb Careful have helped you transform the roundness of your apple figure, and exercise will help you stay that way.

Like me, many of you may have days that seem to get increasingly busy, with longer work days and crazier schedules, so it may sound unreasonable to try to include *one more thing* in your insane schedule. But try to move away from your old line of reasoning and give yourself a new direction. Imagine that by including just a small amount of physical activity, you are actually doing something that will increase your overall energy level.

There are many effective ways to fit movement into your life. We all know about parking our cars farther away from the door. How about parking our bodies farther away by getting off the bus or train sooner or walking three or four or fourteen blocks past your destination and back? You will find that once you get moving, you won't be able to stop! You will soon find that suddenly it's not so hard to get out of bed a few minutes early or that you prefer to use your lunch break to eat a brief meal at your desk, using the rest of the time for a quick walk through the neighborhood. Those of you lucky enough to have a workout space near where you work might become quick-change artists—creatively fitting in a workout during the course of the day. Why wait until the weekend, thinking you'll do a longer workout when you have the time? Make it happen now—the future will take care of itself.

ENDORPHIN RUSH

Endorphins are chemicals released by your brain that basically tell you "You're happy!" They naturally occur when you experience something pleasurable: eating an ice cream cone, having sex with your partner, watching an interesting play, or looking at artwork. Whatever gives you pleasure creates a chemical release that makes you feel good. Exercise does just this for your body. It sends a chemical message to your brain that says "This feels great!"

Exercise has the power to deliver body pleasure by increasing the natural release of endorphins. It's as if you are giving your body a present, and it is giving you a thank-you note—a rush of good feeling that makes you feel more at peace with yourself and sends you a message of reinforcement and encouragement that says, "That was great, now let's do it again!" Once your body—and your mind—get used to this rush of pleasure, you will be hooked into *exercise euphoria*.

KUDOS FOR EXERCISE

As you begin exercising regularly, you will:

- Stretch out those legs and even touch those toes
- Achieve an overall sense of well-being that comes from your body humming instead of plodding along
- Improve your body composition, and you will be creating a leaner, healthier you
- Nurture your noncerebral self
- Have more energy
- Feel more serene
- Experience an endorphin rush
- Invest in a healthier future

MOVING TO YOUR OWN GROOVE

This program doesn't offer a set regimen or a way to exercise. On the contrary, it's designed to fit your needs and lifestyle, as flexible as you soon will be. The truth is, even if you think you hate all types of exercise, it's more likely that you just probably haven't found your niche or given yourself enough time to let it get under your skin. There are a lot more exercise options than just running, biking, or aerobic classes. There are an endless number of enjoyable activities and opportunities. Again, think of what gets you excited and inspired. Did you like to ice skate as a child? Why not take it up again? Or maybe you want something that doesn't require practice. Do you like to spend time outdoors? Well, walking puts you outside. Why not incorporate a morning walk into your routine? That's a great way to start the day. You don't have to walk a mile—around the block is a good beginning. And if you're someone who needs a goal in mind, then maybe make the objective of your walk to buy the morning paper or your afternoon apple snack.

Here are some pointers for creating and sticking to a new exercise program:

- Choose the *type* of exercise that suits you
- Give yourself *alternatives* to keep interested
- Decide on *how often* is enough
- *Schedule* exercise ahead of time
- Choose a *time that makes sense* for you
- *Take the plunge*

WHAT TYPE ARE YOU?

Are you a group exercise person or do you prefer to play solo? If you're a team player, then maybe picking up a tennis racket again and becoming part of a round-robin or joining a volleyball group or paddle tennis group may be a great way of staying healthy. It may also be a wonderful way to meet new friends in a fun-filled environment. You can even do this with walking by creating your own informal walking club, like one of my clients did. If you're like Michael, then you'll prefer working out solo. At age forty-eight, Michael decided he wanted to learn how to row. He'd seen an advertisement in his local paper for a masters rowing team. When he inquired, he discovered that he didn't have to have years of experience; but rather, he could learn as he went along. So he signed up. He borrowed a boat and took a few lessons, and once he felt sturdy enough to manage the boat, he discovered remarkable pleasure in being out on the water by himself. "I've never experienced such serenity before in my life; it's *almost* as good as holding my newborn son in my arms for the first time." Talk about an endorphin rush!

Perhaps you too enjoy singular activities like running or swimming that let you be alone, giving you the time and space to let your other concerns, responsibilities, and worries recede into the background. But you can also learn to relax by working out with others. Once a week, before heading home to his wife and kids, Glen heads to a karate class held in the gym of the local elementary school. "It tests my brain and my body. I feel a little self-conscious sometimes, but I'm getting past that. The training has taught me how to clear my mind and organize my thoughts. At the end of a long day, it works better than a beer!"

THE EXERCISE EXPLORER

Need more of a challenge? If you've been a regular exerciser for years—running, biking, playing tennis, or other racquet sports—you may want to consider checking out these more demanding ways to test your workout mettle:

- ty-bo
- yoga for athletes (Ashtanga, or Power Yoga)
- rock climbing (on the wall at your gym or at your nearest park)
- hiking
- triathalon
- mountain biking
- spin class

DIFFERENT STROKES: GIVE YOURSELF SOME ALTERNATIVES

I have a client who changes his sport each season, not because he competes in the decathlon but because he says he gets bored. From swimming to running to yoga to spinning classes at the gym—he knows himself—he gets bored easily and so he shifts his activities every few months so he won't *not* exercise. Another client just started doing yoga tapes in the morning. "They take only twenty-five minutes and I feel so much more relaxed throughout my day." Sheila says working in her garden feels like exercise—and it is. Charles was used to playing paddle tennis but, after a knee injury, he discovered archery. It may sound arcane and maybe it is, but if it gets you active, then it's good for you!

As with the supplements, there is no one-size-fits-all program for exercise. My pleasure may be your nightmare. Try everything, have fun, and remember you are allowed to enjoy yourself!

WHAT DO YOU MEAN, LADIES DON'T SWEAT?

Sweating can be glamorous. Maybe not if you're on your way to a meeting and you're soaking through your shirt, but next time you're flipping through a magazine—from *Vogue* to *Men's Journal*—notice the new image of a good time: sweat-drenched bodies and smiling faces. Sweating feels great—it's empowering. And it's a way to cleanse the body and get rid of toxins through your body's largest organ, the skin. Talk about a real release!

HOW OFTEN IS ENOUGH?

How much time *should* you exercise? This is up to you. Some of you, especially those of you who already work out regularly, will want to spend a lot of time skating, biking, and playing tennis. And there really is not a limit on how much unless, of course, it begins to remove you from life. But for many of you who are still exercise novices, just try committing two to three days a week to start, spending at least fifteen minutes to work out. You'll be surprised at how you will want to increase this frequency faster than you can imagine. You'll be increasing the time and the days and having fun while you're doing it. Eventually, you'll want to get up to about three to five days a week for, again, at least twenty-five minutes a day—and perhaps eventually up to forty-five. This won't be hard; you're going to love it!

If I had the time, I would exercise every single day, but at different intensity levels. As it is, some days, my workouts are pretty strenuous; other days, they are softer, easier. After a long, tiring day at the office, I like taking a long bike ride, adventuring beyond my neighborhood and heading toward a path that encircles a large bay. When I choose an activity such as biking, it's hard to remember that I am working; it sure doesn't feel like it when I pedal down the quiet street, catching the last ray of light, listening to the birds, and just luxuriating in my own sense of balance and quiet. It may be difficult to measure fully this type of exercise, but it's not hard to imagine the extraordinary benefits when you feel so satisfied. Next time you look wistfully at your bike rather than your gym bag, follow your longing. The pleasure, ease, and sense of freedom will do wonders for your body and soul.

ARE YOU RUNNING AWAY?

Some of you are part of the many men and women who like to take two exercise classes back to back, lift weights four to five times, and make working out a passionate focus of each and every day. But sometimes, this kind of exercising begins to control us instead of being a pleasurable addition to one's daily schedule. Sometimes people can actually use exercise to run away from their problems. I listened to a friend reminisce about her ex-husband, who would spend hours jogging in the neighborhood with his male buddies on weekends, seriously diminishing the time he spent at home. She heard after they had separated that he had traded his addictive running for a much more moderate forty-minute jog several times a week. It didn't take long for my friend, talented psychologist that she is, to realize he was running away from their problems instead of toward them. Just as with overeating, the need for perpetual motion can really be fueled by a need to avoid life's tougher moments.

SCHEDULE EXERCISE AHEAD OF TIME

If you really want to get the most out of the program, then you should schedule exercise just as you would any priority. It's easier to keep a contract than to let days slip loosely by one after the other without ever getting started. I love to plan some exercise for five days of the week. Sometimes I can do more, and sometimes less. I know that I leave very early three days a week to go to my Manhattan office, which makes early morning activity impossible on a Tuesday, Wednesday, or Thursday. (No matter what the benefits of exercise are, they are not strong enough to get me to move at 5:30 A.M.) My exercise those mornings occurs around getting in and out of the shower, bending to dry my feet, and raising my toothbrush in my hand. On these days, I try to get in a lunch-time walk, but that doesn't always happen. But for the rest of the week, I am dedicated to getting in four decent workouts—most of which entail some weight training and a brisk

> Don't forget to hydrate. Water, water, and more water! Keep your body flush before, during, and after exercise.

walk or jog. My work schedule has me walking Friday, Saturday, Sunday, and Monday. If I miss Sunday, then I *know* I *can't* miss Monday.

Recently I signed on for a three-day, sixty-mile walk to benefit breast cancer. Talk about a motivator! I used the race not only as a benchmark to raise money but also to get me back into better condition after slipping for a short period. Perhaps you have a similar motivator in your area. There's nothing like a worthy cause to make us move a bit faster.

GREAT INGREDIENTS FOR A GOOD TIME

Another idea for a great way to exercise that will surely make you feel incredible for the next few weeks is moving your body for a cause. I know how great I felt when I walked alongside three thousand other cancer survivors and supporters with the beautiful Hudson Valley vistas all around us as we raised money for cancer research. It is not just an athletic experience, it's a spiritual one.

WHAT TIME MAKES SENSE?

What's the best time of day to exercise? When you will do it! I like to start the day by doing my almost-daily exercise, a walk or a jog in the neighborhood or on a treadmill. That way, I know that I did it, and I feel wonderful all day, *and* I don't have to get dressed and showered again. Also, even with my good intentions, my day can become very busy and I can become too distracted, or lose the desire when I'm running late for a meeting.

You might get sidetracked by the kids' return from school. If you exercise in the morning, getting it under your belt, you not only feel the physical charge throughout your day but you also feel a sense of accomplishment and what a bonus that is! You know the drill. But again, if you love your afternoons to take that jog, then go for it! Just try to pick a time that you are more likely to stick to.

> ### USE YOUR JOURNAL
>
> Remember to use your journal to record and schedule your exercise.

TAKE THE PLUNGE!

There's a reason I don't even mention exercise in my first one or two meetings with a new client: I know when they achieve Basic Balance, they will feel more ready and able to introduce exercise as part of their routine. If you're one of those people for whom the very word *exercise* conjures up a lot of feelings of dread and anxiety—fear not. I haven't lost one client yet. I want you just to get out there. That's right, just one foot in front of the other. Start off by working out two or three times a week. Sound like a lot? Start with fifteen-minute intervals of riding the stationary bike, walking, or doing the StairMaster. You can do fifteen minutes! Sounds much easier than you thought? Well, it is. And, if you feel up to it, increase it to twenty minutes the next week; before you know it, you will have graduated to forty minutes.

When I first met my husband, Arthur, he seduced me into believing he was a regular jogger—my passion at the time. So on one of our first dates, we went jogging. When he asked how long we were going to run, I said thirty minutes. As we were passing the thirtieth minute, I kept going. After about fifty minutes, Arthur, who was not finding it as easy as he thought, glanced at his watch and declared, "You said a half an hour and time's up!" And so we stopped. That would be the last time he ever stopped looking at his watch.

I soon discovered that though he was a natural athlete, he chose not to do anything physical. In fact, he seemed to make it a practice *not* to overextend himself physically. After several years of being together, I would beg him to go brisk walking with me at night, since I found it vastly improved my disposition after a day inside. Eventually he would come, setting strict limits, and with me insisting we walk a few more blocks. No fool he, he had learned his lesson earlier: We were not allowed to walk thirty-one minutes, one minute beyond the thirty he said he would do. These thirty minutes did not necessarily bring us back home. Many evenings I found myself sitting at the Häagen-Dazs watching him enjoy some dreamy, creamy ice-cream concoction. Sometimes I think he pulled a real Tom Sawyer on me, prematurely ending my nightly entreaty.

Now that was a long time ago, and it was only some years later that Arthur himself found he wanted to exercise. Once he began to roll back his carbs and get into *better balance,* he found he had so much more energy that he began awakening at 6:00 A.M., raring to go. Today he begins his morning with a challenging walk, rounded out by four hundred stomach crunches and moderate weight lifting. Sometimes I have to ask myself, is this the man I married?

Even the smallest increase can make a huge impact. Diane, a fifty-something woman, began the Carb-Careful Solution unable to walk the four blocks from her apartment to her office. When I asked her what type of exercise she preferred, she responded by shrugging her shoulders. Finally she admitted, "I don't remember the last time I exercised. I have so little energy, it's hard to move. I can't even imagine myself doing anything. I am so overweight and my body is so out of shape." After two months, she not only was walking the four blocks to her office, but she had also extended her walk to two miles—an incredible accomplishment for a woman who needed to lose more than one hundred pounds. At her latest visit to my office, she was ecstatic that she had followed my advice and had added free weights to her exercise routine. Unable to work with a trainer, at my recommendation Diane followed a simple program designed by Miriam Nelson in her book *Strong Women Stay Young* and loved it.

Though you may not be in Diane's position, you may relate to her fear of beginning an exercise regimen. I always think of another client, Carol, who had an aversion to exercise because she said she didn't like the way she jiggled when she was in an aerobics class. She felt like a teenager, back in high school when all the other girls seemed to have it together except for her. Now as an adult, she'd look around the workout room of her gym, and all she'd see were other women who seemed to be in so much better shape than she. After months of self-inflicted torment, Carol finally gave up her club membership. "It's too much trouble to get there" was her reason.

Carol and I discussed how the peer pressure she experienced at the gym made her feel intimidated, preventing her from getting in shape and starting a regular workout routine. I was struck once again about how ironic it is that our society has groomed people to get in shape but at the same time discourages them because they don't have the *right shape*!

Carol couldn't believe the changes in her body with even very moderate exercise. Simply doing a half hour on a stationary bike began to improve her metabolism and control her chemistry. By making her body less insulin resistant, she lost weight for the first time in years. "Everyone is raving, telling me that I look incredible. I don't think I'll ever get tired of hearing it, even if it is becoming a little embarrassing." Beyond the weight loss, the resultant improvement in her body composition dramatically redesigned her body into a much trimmer, more attractive shape. Carol quickly joined the ranks of the converted. Like so many others who allow themselves to schedule and commit to an exercise routine, Carol now misses physical activity when she is forced to skip it.

If you're like Diane or Carol, and still at a loss for how to begin to exercise, I suggest you examine what you like to do naturally. For example, when you're alone in the car and your favorite song comes on, do you have the desire to blast it and start dancing?

Well start! Buy a bunch of your favorite CDs, make a tape, and put it on at home. If you don't want the neighbors to watch you, then pull down the shades. Don't feel silly, *this is exercise.* You're getting your heart rate up, you'll probably even break a sweat, and it's fun! Incorporate this into your daily routine, or at least three to five times a week, and you're on your way. Mowing the lawn, washing the windows, almost any household chore can become exercise if you are moving around for a reasonable amount of time. Do you occasionally turn into Ethel-the-cleaning-woman, madly vacuuming the house, dusting every surface, and reorganizing the linen closet? Some of us may think you're crazy, but the three or four hours you spend cleaning or doing yard work are giving you a workout.

Ask yourself these questions:

1. Is your closet crowded with slightly used equipment and clothing for jogging, tennis, bowling, or soccer—hobbies that you thought you'd enjoy but never found the time to do?
2. Do you spend Saturday morning hunting to find out where you dropped your sneakers after last Saturday's basketball game?
3. Do you become evasive if your significant other suggests a walk after dinner?
4. Do you begin your workweek with a stressful search for your keys?
5. Does your temperature rise every time you are stuck in traffic?
6. Do you meditate by munching on corn chips?
7. Is your idea of exercise climbing a step stool to find the chocolate bar you hid from yourself?

Please don't panic: I am not asking you to commit to a lifetime. Just give it a try for four weeks and see how you feel. If after four weeks of slightly increasing either the time or the frequency and you don't love what you're doing, then you can stop with my blessing. But I know you will want to keep exercise in your life, not because I say so but because you will love how you feel. Soon you'll be able to run up the stairs, move with greater ease, and go through your day with an overall sense of well-being. You must rely on yourself. At first, it may feel overwhelming, but it only takes a few good weeks of determination—and for many of you even less than that—and then it suddenly all just comes together.

Exercise does not have to feel like a punishment. Soon it will begin to feel like a joy. As one of my clients, Liza, pointed out, "I can see how the exercise works; you should see my dog, Puck! He thinks he is a puppy again. He is so much better since I am speed walking. He's become so devilish on our morning walks, and he's ten years old." Just wait until Liza realizes that it's not just her dog who is feeling and looking younger.

JUST DO IT!

The hardest part of exercising is making the decision to do it. Once you get started, just a few minutes in, it becomes a done deal and not an effort, at least not a must-I-do-this? punishment.

THE DYNAMICS OF EXERCISE: AEROBIC VS. MUSCLE BUILDING

Although any kind of movement can be considered to be good for your body, there are at least two ways to classify exercise—aerobic and muscle-building. Aerobic exercise is any activity that increases your heart rate. When you regularly raise your heart rate and keep it raised for at least twenty minutes, then you strengthen your heart and lungs. You will feel this strength as you climb the stairs or walk up a hill or carry groceries in from the car. Internally, you are moving oxygen around your bloodstream more efficiently. Walking, running, spinning, cycling, and tennis are aerobic activities that get your blood pumping, the heart beating, and you breathing at a quicker pace. Researchers have found that only twelve minutes a day of aerobic activity for six days a week or twenty-five minutes for three days is enough to increase your metabolic rate. Do keep in mind that you should be able to carry on a conversation during aerobic activity; if you can't speak, then you are probably working too hard and need to slow down or stop and give your body a rest.

GETTING AEROBIC

To calculate your target heart rate, subtract your age from 220 and multiply that number by .75. The answer is the number of beats per minute you should feel when you take your pulse. See chart for average target ranges. These are good safety factors when you are beginning to exercise.

FREE WEIGHTS FOR BETTER BODY COMPOSITION

Strength-building exercise does just that: strengthens the muscles of your body. This is the key to improving your body composition. And as I said above, the more muscle you have, the more fat you burn, which increases insulin receptivity of cells. Your body contains both fat and lean muscle but only lean muscle is capable of burning significant calories. The basic, energy-burning engine of the body is its lean muscle tissue. Like a couch potato, the fat tissue simply sits there, a storage form of energy that the body hoards and doesn't use. Less muscle leads to a slower metabolism, which in a roundabout way worsens your Metabolic Mix-Up. Men tend to be biologically more muscular; so yes, they tend to lose weight faster just because they metabo-

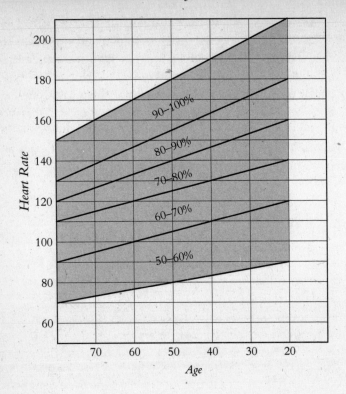

lize faster (I never said this was fair). Another reason to eat reasonable amounts of protein: Only protein can make muscle, and muscle must be made every day.

During my training for the breast cancer walk, I included free weights into my regular workout. Never having used weights before, I began with five-pound weights and gradually increased to ten-pound hand weights. This is an easy way to build muscle, and I loved it. It was hard work but exciting to feel my upper body strength, which had never been very apparent, improve with each passing week. I could actually feel—and see—my body grow stronger.

Muscle-building activity involves exercises that use resistance in pulling, pushing, or lifting. Some easy ways to increase muscle mass using resistance are:

• Add light hand or ankle weights when you walk. Three- or five-pound weights are a good choice for most women; men can use eight to ten pound weights.

• Use the force of gravity against your body for resistance by doing leg lifts, sit-ups, or push-ups. Working the larger muscles in your legs will increase your total muscle mass the fastest. Using ankle weights or rubber bands during leg lifts will give you even greater resistance.

• Do lunges as you talk on the phone, watch television, or are waiting for the water to boil for your veggies.

• Lift up on your toes while you are standing at work, while doing dishes, or while folding clothes.

LARGER MUSCLES BURN MORE FAT

According to Dr. Cheryle Hart, "There is no direct way to get rid of fat in any particular area of the body. Sit-ups may firm your stomach but will not increase muscle mass quickly. The best way to trim your waist is to activate your larger muscle groups such as the thigh and buttock muscles. Working these muscles increases your body's overall metabolism and speeds up fat burning."

TIP: BE FAIR TO YOUR BODY

Be sure to alternate areas of your body. It's best not to work the same muscles two days in a row because muscles need time to recover. Instead, alternate: Work your legs one day and your upper body the next day.

THE SLOW BURN

When it rains or I have an early morning meeting, I avoid feeling disappointed by replacing my morning walk with brisk, short walks down the hallways throughout the workday. Even this little jump start for your body will add some spark to your day. Check out the spark you can ignite with various activities:

Calorie Burning Guide

Activity	15 min	30 min	45 min	60 min
Aerobics (high impact)	165	320	500	660
Aerobics (low impact)	135	270	400	540
Basketball (game playing)	140	280	430	550
Baseball/Softball	92	159	240	317
Circuit Training (with weights)	185	320	455	580
Cycling (6 mph)	75	130	190	240
Cycling (12 mph)	100	200	300	410
Cycling (15 mph)	150	320	480	600
Cross-Country Skiing	145	300	450	600
Dancing (swing)	110	205	293	390
Dancing (line)	65	138	195	258
Downhill Skiing	100	200	300	400
Football	140	280	390	530
Golf (Walking)	45	115	170	230
Golf (carrying clubs)	80	170	260	340
Handball	165	325	490	655

Activity	15 min	30 min	45 min	60 min
Hiking (average incline)	105	190	280	360
Hockey	142	290	420	555
Horseback Riding (general)	65	130	195	260
Ice Skating (general)	110	225	340	445
In-line Skating	150	300	450	600
Jump Rope	170	290	460	620
Kayaking	75	150	225	300
Martial Arts	180	328	485	645
Racquetball	110	225	340	450
Rock Climbing (ascending)	192	388	540	722
Rowing Machine	150	350	475	650
Running (10-min mile pace)	180	360	540	730
Running (8-min mile pace)	225	450	670	925
Sex (average pace)	24	49	75	97
Ski Machine	125	280	425	575
Stair Climber	155	310	460	618
Swimming (freestyle)	130	250	380	510
Tennis (singles)	110	225	350	450
Volleyball	48	90	144	190
Walking (flat, 17-min mile pace)	65	130	200	275
Walking (hills, 17-min mile pace)	90	180	260	380
Water Aerobics	70	140	210	280
Weeding a Garden	90	160	230	320
Weight Training	130	270	385	510

Activity	15 min	30 min	45 min	60 min
Wrestling (5-min match)	115	180	290	387
Yoga	70	120	185	240

AN ENDLESS SUMMER

The benefits of exercise are endless: Exercise increases the rate of metabolism, strengthens heart and cardiovascular systems, and improves your body composition. And what a bonus: The more oxygen to your brain, the more clear and quick your mind works. In general, when you exercise, your body functions better overall. You don't have to do a lot for positive change to occur: Walk fifteen minutes per day and you will notice a difference, not only just a loss of weight and reshaping of your body but you will also feel better!

If this isn't enough incentive to add exercise to your daily/weekly routine, consider this fact: The great majority of cancer patients have lived sedentary lives and while I don't like to scare you, it scares *me* if I can't get you to move. The research shows that all of us with the Metabolic Mix-Up are more vulnerable to developing prostate or breast cancer.

The incredible boost in energy you will get from exercise will convince you even more. Before Tom got into a regular exercise routine, he often felt tired. He noticed that his energy had increased as he started the Carb-Careful Solution but not as much or as fast as he would have liked. But when he added the half-mile walk to work twice a week, he noticed the difference almost immediately. "I felt so much more full of life! I became a convert—now no one can interfere with this part of my day."

He became so inspired by this boost in energy that he started to walk to work *every* day. He told me, "I not only feel physically better, but I also feel mentally better than I have in ages." Have you ever heard of a runner's high? Well, Tom was experiencing the same phenomenon. He is a living example of what scientific research has proven: that exercise can actually help decrease depression in people who suffer from it. Now Tom is so hooked that he uses his weekends as an opportunity for even longer walks, instead of crashing on the couch to catch up on spectator sports.

DON'T FLAKE OUT

On weekends, people have a tendency to flake out on their exercise because they don't have the schedule of their weekdays to keep them focused. Don't use the weekends as a time to veg out, becoming a couch potato in front of your television. Instead, challenge yourself to do a longer or more intense workout on the weekend when you have more time—to enjoy it and to relax afterward.

CHECKLIST FOR EXERCISE

1. Have you checked with your doctor before beginning a new exercise program?
2. Are you committed? If you are not already a regular exerciser, make the decision and consciously resolve to add exercise into your weekly routine.
3. Are you scheduling your exercise in advance? Decide on Sunday what days you are going to exercise that week so you plan ahead. If you don't plan ahead, you're more likely not to do it. Then you can always change. By writing it down, you help reinforce your commitment.
4. Are you describing your exercise in your journal? Try by adding a section or room for exercise notes in your journal. Write down how it feels during and after the exercise—I guarantee that in a few weeks you will not believe your own handwriting.

THE SECRET SIDE OF EXERCISE

When you look at exercise from an anthropological point of view, you'll see that humans were designed to move, not to be sedentary as so many of us are in today's culture. Our early ancestors' very survival depended on it. From the days of hunting and gathering, men and women were always moving—to collect the firewood and the food and to escape predators. But in our modern culture, with all of our modern shortcuts, we have lost this natural way to exercise. In its stead, we have created many time-saving devices—and for what, really? To spend more time listlessly sitting in front of the TV. This is not a judgment call on my part, I love watching *West Wing* just as much as you. But we have to remember that if we disregard our biological need to move, we are in a sense neglecting our spiritual center; it is no wonder that feelings of sadness are replaced with hope when we get going.

Exercise should be enjoyable, easy, and energizing—so let's get started! Do it! Enjoy it! And whatever you do, don't think of it as gym class. For heaven's sake, I encourage you to smile at the gym junkies, after all you share the secret—the secret of exercise.

PART THREE

Your Life's Endless Rainbow

—∞∞∞—

CHAPTER 9

Mind Games

Transforming Attitudes That Shape Eating Habits

THE FOOD CONNECTION

The power of foods cannot be underestimated. This fact became clear yet again, when after the World Trade Center disaster, one of my clients, Pamela, a successful media executive, arrived at my office feeling very vulnerable and highly emotional, quite close to being totally demoralized. She had been doing and feeling remarkably well on the program up until this time. But the weekend following the horrible attack, she returned home to see her family. Over the weekend, she had proceeded to eat every sugar-laden treat she could fit into her newly slender body. As she shakily recalled, "Before the tragedy, I had been feeling extraordinary—just extraordinary—doing the steps. But this past week I've been a mess. The world news is tearing me apart. So when I went home, I had all my favorite comfort foods: homemade breads, pies, and cookies. Once I start, I can't stop. It's almost as though I were possessed—possessed by a force stronger than my sense of reason. It becomes so easy to convince myself that since I have ruined the day, why bother to stop! So I just continue eating." She paused, and then said, "This thing you keep saying— that I'm a Sugar Baby—well the only way I do without it is to agree that my connection to sugar rules my life." Pamela and I talked about how, instead of going for sugar, she should nurture herself on the weekend, give herself something that would comfort her, such as a massage or a good movie. She came in the following week, understandably still upset, but considerably better. She was now better able to cope with stressful situations as they arose. She had heard my message. She had also regained her spirit. "I know we had talked about giving myself something nice—well, I didn't have the time. But I decided to get my foods under control and that felt better than any massage I could get." When you're feeling out of control, you are out of control! When imbalanced blood sugar sits in the driver's seat, you need more than a seat belt to stay on board!

Everyone has a relationship with food, and often this relationship is well formed even in childhood. Most of us develop powerful emotional connections to the foods we eat and the way in which we eat them. And as Pamela's story shows, these connections can often be negative in some way. Who dives into a pint of ice cream after an argument with a friend or colleague? Who begins fantasizing about dinner in the middle of a tense business meeting? Oh you poor boy, are you hurt? Here's a cookie! Many of us rely on food as a comfort. And while there are many wonderful things about food—it is delicious, nurturing, pleasurable, and even tantalizing—there can be a too-strong connection between food and emotions. When food becomes the drug of choice and the main way to soothe confusing or disturbing feelings, then an unhealthy dependence on eating as a way out can develop.

For those of us with the Metabolic Mix-Up, our connection to food is greater, the love affair stronger. Like many people, we learned to use food as a substitute for or an extension of real feelings, but the way we use food has an even stronger impact. Our chemical reaction to the carbohydrates, particularly sugar, is much more intense, almost manic in behavior. Remember my walk home from school on Fridays? The creamy doughnut, the delectable cake? The engraving of my connection to sweets went deeper because my body's reaction was so much greater. And if dessert was withheld because of some minor infraction, I was beyond disappointed; I was thrown into despair. I needed that hit.

With this kind of shared history, it should be no surprise to those of us with the Metabolic Mix-Up that when we start unearthing these old eating patterns and begin to change how we eat and think about food that our whole world feels suddenly shaky. There is no doubt about it. Changing your lifestyle and diet is part physical, part emotional.

When we eat food instead of dealing with our feelings directly, we are listening to what our bodies need, but we are hearing the wrong message. As a result, we usually end up eating our feelings. When you combine this behavior with someone who is insulin resistant, then the challenge to control your foods to feel better and assure vital health becomes a battle of the wills: your will against that of your chemistry.

Think of how babies learn to soothe and calm themselves: They begin to put their little fists in their mouths, eventually finding their thumbs. But parents often give babies pacifiers, and the children learn to calm themselves by sucking on a treat, something outside of themselves. When a child learns to rely too much on a pacifier, they don't learn alternative ways to settle down and relax within themselves. And when they are too old to whip out a pacifier, they turn to food, something available and tasty to push into their mouths.

Reaching and maintaining balanced blood sugar will give you the greatest and most lasting comfort available. Once you have your blood sugar under control, you not only tame the wild call of your Sugar Baby but you are also better able to handle the distractions, stresses, and challenges of everyday life. Stress is ever present in our lives, and I have not yet met the person who has managed to live a stress-free life, no matter how Zen-like they may be. I meditate every morning, so believe me, I appreciate and know firsthand its power to calm the body and mind. But if blood sugar is not controlled, then all the mantras, all the yoga positions in the world won't work to help you live your life. Blood sugar is like a tidal wave, able to take up everything in its path. And our best defense is to be balanced, ready to handle and manage stress instead of having it manage us.

We've been talking about learning to rethink your approach to food and its impact on your body. As your new routine becomes more familiar, and you become more at ease with the Carb-Careful Solution, you will find that this becomes the way you eat. And when you don't eat this way, it will be the exception, not the rule. Yet often inside the most well-intentioned of us something happens that somehow gets between us and success. One client of mine recently encountered a threat to her hard-won serenity and peace of mind. Beth is a middle-aged production manager at an investment firm. Recently her company had laid off a significant number of employees. Although Beth felt lucky to keep her job, she soon became overwhelmed because she was expected to assume more responsibility as a result of the loss of workers.

She'd been doing beautifully on the program up until this time, eating on time and in reasonable amounts for her. But after six weeks, she began to retrench. She'd be Carb-Careful one week and the next week, she'd eat pasta for lunch two days in a row, creating a roller-coaster cry for more carbs that would send her blood sugar soaring before its inevitable dive. She was not only fueling her mix-up, but priming it for a starring encore performance after a wonderful, but short, opening run.

When we talked about what was happening, she referred to herself as stupid and her behavior as juvenile, but she felt powerless to stop the destructive eating. It was only when I asked her what would happen if she ate right, how would she feel? She lost no time in telling me that she was terrified—absolutely terrified—that people at work would expect even more from her if she got stronger. "I don't think I can do it. I can't take on more work—I am not sure I can do the job I am supposed to be doing now. I walk around so stressed that I'm on the verge of tears all the time; it's obvious to everyone! I must appear so fragile that they treat me as if I am an invalid. But if I get better, then I'm afraid they will ask me to do even more work!"

I think she was as surprised as I was. Until this point, she'd had no idea that her fear of taking on more work was preventing her from eating well and getting better. She had convinced herself that a stronger, calmer Beth would surely invite demands and pressures that she didn't think she could handle.

Once she touched some of these thoughts and feelings, she realized that she had been living behind a curtain of fear, a wall of resistance that stopped her from living in that calmer, more balanced way. By putting one foot in front of the other, she picked up the pieces of the program. As she became calmer, stronger, and less fragile, she also became more capable. But the irony of it all was that she began to realize she could actually handle the extra work with more ease. Recently she said to me, "Finally I'm able to make this work. I had no idea that my fears were working behind the scenes, causing me to destroy the emotional and physical strength I so badly need." She'd crossed over and was now able to embrace true health.

A GENTLE REMINDER ABOUT BALANCED BLOOD SUGAR

Controlling your chemistry will help you:

- Manage stress more easily
- Feel less tired, more energetic
- Head off high blood pressure
- Lift yourself away from the path to type 2 diabetes

If that was not enough, I often think about writing a book called *Joie de Vivre*, an entire volume dedicated to showing you the way you are supposed to be, the magical promise of balanced blood sugar!

YOU'RE A WORK-IN-PROGRESS

Making the Carb-Careful Solution a part of your everyday life asks you to treat yourself as if you matter and deserve to take care of yourself. And learning to both nurture and nourish yourself is a drive toward optimal health. Don't worry about how you are going to do this. One of my clients, Cindy, who works as a receptionist, had been doing very well on the diet. Diagnosed with high blood pressure and type 2 diabetes, Cindy came to see me because she wanted to get off her medications and feel better. After just a week and a half doing Basic Balance, she began to experience significant improvement. She said to me, "Even my family sees a change. They are telling me that I'm not so jumpy anymore. I don't know whether to be insulted or overjoyed." She chose the joy because balanced blood sugar is like a compass, pointing you in the direction of good feelings.

Then suddenly, she missed an appointment and chose to schedule a phone session instead of coming in person. Speaking with Cindy confirmed something was amiss. In spite of her repeated declarations of good feelings, it was almost as though she were trying to reassure me that she was doing fine. I was not surprised to learn that she hadn't really been keeping her journal, another sign that she was not eating right. When I asked her to fill me in on the meals she was eating, she admitted that she had been less than perfect. Not making time to have her snacks during the workday and waiting too late to eat lunch, she had upset her Basic Balance and was beginning to crave again. She was certainly not in the chemical condition to continue into Carb-Careful. She had not even been able to go food shopping. How could she eat right without the right foods in her refrigerator?

Sometimes forgetting appointments and avoiding in-person contact signal me that the client has not done as well as they would like. Feeling failed, people become less willing to look at how they've been managing on the program. When this happens, it is often necessary to remind them that they are in charge and that the program is something *for them.* Don't let this happen to you. If you have had a problem, don't be concerned. You can always restore your balance by returning to Basic Balance. Just remember: The program always works; you just need to do it.

I had known Cindy was not doing the program correctly. If she had been doing it right, she would be excited, saying, "I can't believe how incredible I feel," instead of just telling me she felt better. And her family would be saying, "We can't believe the difference in you" instead of merely remarking on subtle changes. To people like Cindy I say, "I'm very happy that you're okay and that you're enjoying yourself, but I want more for you. Don't stop because you feel better than terrible. Let's go for great!"

Keep in mind that the diet works in stages, and there is no all or nothing. You're *always* on the program. If you feel you've gotten off track for a few days or even a week or so, then don't disappear into your disappointment at feeling failed. Just stop, become aware of exactly what you need to do, and go back to Basic Balance or make adjustments as needed. Like Mozart getting stuck in the middle of composing a concerto, you too are a work in progress.

Taking care of yourself can feel like the hardest thing you've ever done. But by doing what's best for you, you will discover the power to become the ultimate explorer of life, discovering vast new continents of energy within yourself.

SELFISH VS. SELFLESS

If you feel it is selfish to take time for yourself, then think about the opposite of selfish: selfless, which means having no self at all. Perhaps you need to be a little more selfish in order to be well. You alone can give yourself permission to treat yourself right. Remember, no one can take this from you.

WHAT ARE YOU FEELING?

You may be finding out that embracing the idea of health and truly committing to making important changes is often a subtle, difficult process. Did you notice a big shift in how you felt as you moved from Basic Balance to Carb-Careful? Has increasing your exercise allowed you to handle a few more carbs? Do the supplements give you more flexibility and freedom to try different foods without triggering your insulin resistance? Learning how to identify the foods that make you react is a necessary part of the process, but sometimes you also have to become conscious of how you are *using* food. Sometimes food can be a teddy bear, something to hug and comfort you when you are down. In the coming weeks, as you get more involved in letting go of your chemical connections, it will be important to really examine *why* you eat. Do you use food when you need a hug? What are you feeling? Let the thoughts come. Are you remembering a past love or feeling sad because you have no one new in your life? What about your daily surroundings? Is the unexciting environment dulling your shine? Or perhaps like Beth you are grounding yourself, weighing yourself down with food so that you can't begin to meet new challenges or make difficult transitions. Many of us can feel frustrated with different areas of our lives. This is when we tend to *eat* instead of *feel* our feelings. This tendency to use food as an emotional replacement creates a negative field of downward energy. It usually means we have a negative attitude toward food. Yes, the food may provide momentary comfort, but after you eat your way through a chocolate cake, do you feel any better? Not really. Underneath the comfort lies unspoken powerful, negative connections to food that may be holding you back from truly owning the program.

Use the following checklist to see how you are feeling. By identifying and recognizing thoughts and feelings associated with food, you will stop any attitudes that may be getting between you and working the steps.

1. Is achieving a younger biological self high on your to-do list?
2. Are you committed to doing some work to change how you feel?
3. Do you believe that you can take charge of your health?
4. Are you really ready to change your life or has some frightening test result given you temporary impetus?
5. Do you no longer think about when you can get off the program?
6. Do you no longer believe that being able to change your eating style will take nothing short of moving a mountain?
7. Does your emotional state no longer dictate whether you can be Carb-Careful or not?
8. Are you interested in this investment in your future, or are you just interested in being a short-term trader, just losing some quick weight?
9. Do you feel you can always do better, or do you believe you have it as good as it gets?
10. Does food no longer seem more powerful than you?

If you answer no to any one of these, then you need to pay closer attention to how your feelings toward food may be getting in the way of your success at working the steps of the program. Check your attitude. The best way to keep from getting sidetracked and losing your focus is to stay in touch with how you're feeling. Separate your feelings from your food: If you're feeling depressed or bluesy, go see a movie or rent one. Recently Arthur and I had a week where we had to deal with some upsetting events and we knew we needed an emergency fix. We found it by watching the funniest, most ridiculous movie in the neighborhood.

If you're feeling cranky or out of sorts, a walk around the block or taking a ride for a change of scene can shake you out of your mood. Soaking in a bath laced with relaxing lavender oil might ease those bad feelings inside. Go bowling or play racquetball. Think of what makes you happy aside from those candy bars or milk shakes, and go there. Learn to redirect your mind away from food as the only way to comfort or nurture yourself.

Writing in your journal also helps to reveal both your conscious and unconscious feelings. Transferring your feelings in ink onto the pages of your journal helps you to stay present and accountable, taking the power out of the feelings themselves. As you probably have discovered in other areas of your life, you need to identify the problem before you can make a lasting change.

This new way of eating will change your life, so of course you are going to feel tremors and shifts, both subtle and obvious. Know that changes lie ahead, changes that will enhance your life. Look forward to them with excitement and joy. You will soon be experiencing the incredible benefits of a more vibrant, satisfying, and joyful life. Know that you're almost there—soon you will be walking the four steps as if they were second nature.

CHAPTER 10

Owning the Program

MAKING THE CARB-CAREFUL SOLUTION YOUR OWN

This chapter is about owning the diet. It's about taking the program with you where you go, whenever you go, for however long you are on the go. The Carb-Careful Solution is a program that moves with you, lives with you, breathes with you. As you walk the steps, you are trading one lifestyle for another. You will get used to this way of living; it becomes the way you eat not the exception but the rule. It's versatile, transportable, and malleable—a way of life that can go with you anywhere and doesn't require an endless array of hard-to-find foods. If you have a particularly hard week and have *lost it* a little, don't worry! This does not mean you're off the diet. There is no off or on the diet, you're either eating well or having some trouble. You can always take back the program. Keep going until you're back in better balance. The program always works. You just have to do it. I want to help you make it part of your daily life so much so that you get to a point where you are no longer thinking about it, when thinking ahead about what foods you're going to eat becomes automatic—a flash in your brain like second nature. Sure you do have to give a little thought to what you're going to be eating but in the same way you may plan what you're going to wear or remind yourself to bring your toothbrush, small enough dues for so large a return. Yes, it is possible to take care of yourself when you are not at home. You will be able to take the Carb-Careful Solution on all occasions, including

- when you work
- when you travel
- at a dinner party
- at a restaurant
- when you're sick
- when you're craving carbs

WHEN YOU WORK

Never leave home without it: *breakfast,* of course. Do not become distracted, focused only on getting out of the house on time. You must, absolutely must, fortify yourself against the challenges of the workday. The workplace can be risky territory, filled with pitfalls and temptations. With food all around you, the challenge to stay out of trouble begins right away. Walking past the coffee and bagels in the front office becomes impossible unless you have kept your Basic Balance by having an early breakfast at home. If you just can't face the refrigerator during your morning rush, you must eat breakfast on your way to work if that doesn't mean two hours after you've gotten up.

But for many of you, the snacks that you usually eat at work are often what you rely on to get you through the day. Do you wind up with your hand in your neighbor's cookie stash or do you make frequent trips to the vending machine? Do you find yourself clocking the time until the coffee-klatch hour when coffee's not the only thing that's plentiful? Take Margaret, for instance, who downs three mugs of coffee while chatting with her co-workers, or Terry, who inhales a bagel from the platter placed on the table in the conference room. How can you get through the maze of food challenges at work?

Learn to think ahead. It will become second nature after a while. Don't wait for the morning scramble to get your food together. And don't think you'll make a pit stop on your way to the office. We both know that will never happen. The night before, after dinner, make sure you have the ingredients for your lunch (if you bring your lunch to work) and set aside your Hard Chew snacks. A good shortcut: It's easy to set up three days' worth of snacks by placing them in little plastic baggies—only the veggies and fruit. Add the companion proteins the night before. This way you will be less likely to be caught without your morning and afternoon snacks. I usually have three fully packed baggies standing up in the refrigerator ready to be called into action. It never hurts to bring an extra snack—for that late day or unexpected quick fix.

Take a look at your food journal. Try to introduce some variety. If you don't want to be bored, don't be boring.

Being physically prepared will help you be mentally prepared, allowing you to break old patterns. If at 11:00 A.M. you're used to buying another doughnut from the vending machine, you can now reach for your Hard Chew snack because it'll be right in front of you. If you are in Basic Balance, you not only control the urge for something sweet or starchy but you also continue to benefit from the balance you feel. Remember those decimal points? How $15,500 became $155 with a simple shift of two little decimal places to the left? You can see how such a small move impacts the value of what you can achieve. This is all that it takes to shift your eating habits on a daily basis, and who wouldn't prefer $15,500 to $155? Your food is your decimal point: Keep it in place, and you will be much richer when you don't have to reach for that Krispy Kreme.

If you feel confident and relaxed when you reach for your snack, unembarrassed by your bag of goodies, then it won't be long before your co-workers will want to know what you are doing and if they can have a veggie or two. Some of my busiest and most visible clients have no problem whipping out their baggies filled with cucumbers and celery. One client of mine was even photographed for a national magazine as he was eating an apple, his midmorning Hard Chew snack. Talk about owning the program! He's confident about his choice for good health. He keeps focused on this goal just as he keeps focused on all parts of his life, and most important, he doesn't let what other people think get in his way of feeling well.

Situations at work can develop that seem to disrupt the timing of your snacks—last minute meetings, bosses dropping by for a chat, or perhaps you get stuck in a long meeting and you know it's time for a snack. It's always better to have your snack before the meeting even if this means having it earlier. This will buy you time, as much as three hours in the afternoon when you will be engrossed and unable to break away. If long meetings are a constant in your life, or part of your job description, then stay prepared. Keep your snacks with you or quietly excuse yourself and take a walk toward your office or cubicle, eating on your way. No one knows what you are doing. Remember, it's not more work than it's worth. When you stay in better balance, your focus and performance are enhanced, allowing you to think quickly on your feet all day. Yes, it's that important to keep your blood sugar levels good. I always tell clients that they will *feel* the remarkable impact of the good blood sugar. It won't just be me telling them about the benefits of eating more frequently—they will discover an extraordinary vitality. The outcome of staying balanced is the biggest strength of the program.

HEAD OFF THE HABIT

You'll be getting rid of the bad chemistry; now it's time to get rid of the habit.

WHEN YOU TRAVEL

Part of the excitement of traveling, whether it is for business or pleasure, is that it is a time to try different restaurants, cuisines—particularly if we're going to a foreign country. Yes, you can travel with the Carb-Careful Solution. My clients have taken the program with them to Europe, Asia, and Chicago. Remember you can eat almost anywhere. There are plenty of choices on most menus that are fine for you to order. You will always have the freedom to eat in any bistro in Paris or three-star restaurant in San Francisco. Just keep thinking "combination, combination, combination" and don't forget your supplements. Though your vitamins are not *permission pills,* they will supply some freeing forgiveness as you navigate the culinary terrain of restaurants as you travel.

If you're going to a foreign country, educate yourself on what kinds of food are popular in that country. Unless you're going to a third-world country, you will find fruits and veggies galore. I know when I am in Italy, for example, it's much easier to eat out because Italians just naturally seem to eat well. Italian restaurants also offer much more reasonable portions—what a relief! In fact, you'll find this throughout much (but not all) of Western Europe, and not surprisingly, the people reflect this healthy diet—slimmer men and women and a vibrant-looking older population. If avoiding pasta seems like cruel and unusual punishment while in Rome, then make sure you don't do quite as the Romans do. Wait as long as you can into the trip, and delay the pasta until the evening meal. If you include veggies and protein along with the pasta, not making it the star of the meal, followed by your supplements, then you can enjoy yourself without too much damage.

Sugar Babies may not escape the seduction of a country such as France with its delectable pastries—mouthwatering *pain au chocolat* or croissants—then be sure to rely on your four-star medley, which will help you avoid your typical high reaction to sugar.

By doing some mental preparation such as reading the food section of your guidebook, you can avoid being seduced by some high-trigger foods that will take you days from which to recover. Another way to control the urge to splurge is by travelling prepared. Bring along some Hard Chew snacks that you've packed in plastic bags. If immigration rules allow, bring more snacks than you think you'll need for a day or two. Include an emergency pop-top can of tuna or some other quality protein. You never know when you will be delayed. This way, you won't have to scramble to buy these foods as soon as you arrive. You will be settled in long before you need some reinforcements.

Flexibility is a state of being. Don't panic if you can't find the perfect meal—just try to be reasonable. Most of my clients look forward to an important evening meal. I think you will agree that this is the preferred time to include some glamorous, high-trigger foods if you would like. It's always better to start out the day eating well, saving those shot-out-of-the cannon carbs until evening, being sure to accompany them with proteins whenever possible. Use what you've learned. When it's dinnertime, you are in a much better place to indulge in that fabulous three-course meal since you will soon be safe in your bed, where the backlash cannot be so disturbing.

Vacation or travel time is often an excuse for us to let go and change our typical routine. There is nothing unreasonable about wanting a break; we all deserve rewards and R and R is essential. But don't use this break in your normal routine to drop off the edge, upsetting your chemistry, inviting the insulin resistance to take control and destroy your health!

AT A DINNER PARTY

No one wants to make a fuss at a dinner party. You've known what it feels like to have a guest suddenly announce they've become a vegetarian when your main dish is leg of lamb. No one wants to be the demanding dinner party guest who doesn't get invited back. But there are tricks to the trade even here. I often eat a Hard Chew, adding a companion protein, before I go out, and still join everyone else when dinner is served. This way, I can be there, eating with my friends, without triggering a metabolic roller-coaster ride. Since many dinner parties mean eating late—often past 8:00 or 9:00—you should prevent interrupting your balance by automatically adding a small amount of your protein to the later afternoon snack. This is not to fill your stomach but to keep you in balance. I have a number of Persian clients whose culture insists on eating very late dinners—many past 11:00 P.M. I recommend that they eat a minidinner with a Hard Chew before the party so that they stay in balance. Then they can decide to have veggies and a reasonable amount of protein with their friends later in the evening if they wish. And watch those hors d'oeuvres! Be selective: Some of the most tantalizing are the ones with doughy little trigger carbs wrapped around protein that will have you looking like a puff pastry too! Of course, you may be lucky to find hors d'oeuvres that include some veggies and a protein. Head for those; they are friends to your chemistry.

Social drinking can be a challenge for some people. Here are some tips to keep in mind so that alcohol doesn't sabotage your balance: Avoid drinking right away, and instead of accepting the offered sweet mixed drink or glass of wine, start the evening with a glass of seltzer or mineral water with lime or lemon, telling yourself you will have a drink later if you still wish. It's usually easier to delay instead of saying no. Then if you want to have a glass of wine with dinner, the effect of the sugar will be less reactive. Keep in mind that this is one of those occasions when you may need to increase your supplements in preparation (see Chapter Seven for specific directions). Any social event can be both enjoyable and safe if you simply keep your eye on the prize: a glowing, healthy, joyful you.

> ### DON'T BE SHY
>
> One of the happy changes that I have seen over the years is a new awareness among restaurateurs, who seem to be more open to the health concerns of customers. Both chefs and servers at restaurants are much more accepting and amenable to making changes to a dish if a customer makes a specific request. So don't be shy! Ask for the change that will keep you happy.

AT A RESTAURANT

It's easy to fantasize that New York is like one giant smorgasbord, offering food East Side to West Side, Harlem to Wall Street. Four out of five clients come in with the nervous announcement that they "eat out almost every night." And for some, it's almost every meal. I have to tell them that everyone is eating out a lot. It's not a problem. I reassure my clients that eating out doesn't have to be a trap. Eating at a restaurant, like eating on a plane or when you travel, can still be a pleasurable experience. You just need to follow the rules and walk the steps. And remember to be reasonable: Always include a high-quality protein, as much fiber as possible, and, of course, lots of pure-power veggies. Remember too that American restaurants—big or small, fancy or simple—are notorious for offering huge portions. But they are also becoming flexible. Think about choosing to have a salad and two or three appetizers instead of a main dish. Opening your mind to different ways of ordering will give you freedom that enables you to be more flexible and versatile in what you eat. Still, I cannot deny that eating out can trigger the food sensualist in even the most disciplined of us.

First, be careful not to go to dinner in a carb-crazy state. You will begin to notice that even your favorite restaurant already offers wonderful, varied choices from pure-power lists, as well as the middle road. You might just have to ask the server to vary a dish or leave something off the plate without doing an imitation of Meg Ryan's character in *When Harry Met Sally.* You can be reasonable at even the most unlikely restaurants, although Mexican and Indian can present special problems. You may have to make some adjustments to what the menu offers but the problem remains that unless you are prepared to allow in a reactive food, these restaurants can be more challenging than some of the many other places from which you can choose. If you make the decision that you've done without your Mexican food long enough and choose to indulge in a high-trigger food such as enchiladas, you can lessen the impact if you eat it in the company of high-quality proteins and veggies and buffer it by ongoing supplements. It's not that I recommend submerging yourself and leaving your carb-careful state, but I am a realistic food sensualist—the perfect combination for knowing what will come up, what is doable, and what is too depriving.

Never eat other people's food. If you are going to challenge your chemistry, let it be something you want, not something someone else wants you to have. If you're at a restaurant with friends or business associates and you feel some pressure to join in either wine or a beer with the meal, you can always learn how to decline gracefully without bringing too much attention to yourself. Use my delay tactic, and when you're asked whether you'd like a drink, smile and say, "Not just now, maybe later," putting your guest at ease while giving him the freedom to do what he wants. When later comes, most people are no longer riveted to whether you will drink or not, and you have managed to keep your blood sugar intact.

WHEN YOU'RE SICK

Being sick can sometimes catapult us back into childhood, giving us an excuse to go carb crazy as we look to comfort ourselves and indulge in foods that make us feel warm and cozy. And when you want to be taken care of, visions of sugarplums will dance in your head. Having the mix-up, your sickness-induced fantasies will not be about the lullabies you used to hear or a mother who used to rub your back and check your vital signs. Your fantasies more than likely will be about all the wonderful comfort foods (aka carbohydrates) that your visiting friends can bring you. When I was a child, the standard sick fare was toast with jelly. While I am no longer interested in toast with jelly, feeling sick still conjures up thoughts of the starchy sweet surprises of those early years.

Try to battle the sick blues by working the steps of the program. If you can, try to keep your proteins in place. And even if you don't feel like eating a lot, a small amount at a reasonable time will protect you from sinking too deep and triggering your insulin insult.

Of course, you should nurture yourself when you're sick. Buy yourself some extra magazines to leaf through or snuggle under your favorite blanket, and by all means, allow yourself to take that nap. Giving yourself these special treats is some of the strongest medicine there is—more powerful and lasting than your most familiar comfort foods. Getting your comfort from a healthy place can be a lifesaver in many ways. Researchers have found that elderly people who have pets actually live longer in a two-way relationship: The pets nurture their owners and their owners nurture their pets. But always return to the key way to restore your balance: Keeping your chemistry under control ensures a wonderful state of well-being and lasting comfort—sick or well.

WHEN YOU'RE CRAVING CARBS

You've loved them—no, craved them—your whole life. It's understandable that every once in a while you will choose them again. Remember, there is room to allow your favorite foods—maybe it's as simple as a side of french fries. Just deal with it: Watch the amount and be reasonable. Try to forget the ketchup but not the companion protein and veggie. One of my clients always fantasizes about Häagen-Dazs ice cream in bed. That's the combo that sends her to the moon. At first she tried to negotiate with me by promising to have low-fat ice cream. I told her it's better to satisfy her fantasy rather than go only half way. Sometimes you need to have food that is good for your soul. I just don't want you to crave it. Be selective. By knowing that you can have an occasional, reasonable amount of your sweet or starchy trigger foods, these foods no longer have the power to hold you at their mercy.

When you start making excuses to look for more, you'll know you've awakened the sleeping giant. And if you have a particularly difficult week, don't worry, just keep plugging! This does not mean you're off the diet. Don't give up. There is no on or off the diet; you are always doing the best you can. You are just eating more or eating less, so drop the guilt instead of the diet. No one can take this away from you. It will take only a few days to get your blood sugar under control with Basic Balance. This first step is always there and available to you. As you live on the Carb-Careful Solution, you will go longer and longer without having a problem, and when a problem does arise, you will be able to fix your foods immediately. In no time at all, such slips will become the exception rather than the rule.

The Carb-Careful Solution can move with you, follow you, be with you. It's your match made in heaven. You simply need to learn to think about foods in a different way, training yourself to eat in a reasonable way. Taking a few minutes to think ahead about how you will negotiate when you travel, go to work, to a restaurant as you live your life will help you be prepared to keep yourself in balance. Soon you'll feel like you've been eating this way your entire life: It simply becomes what you do.

TIPS FOR EVERYDAY LIFE

On your road to joie de vivre, keep these tips in mind:

• Examine your food diary (your journal) to see if you slipped up anywhere. Have you written down everything? What about that Milky Way Light that followed you out of the grocery store? What about the ketchup that slipped onto your burger? By writing in your journal, you stay connected to paying attention to what you are eating, reminding yourself to use food as decimal points placed for higher value.

• Think ahead. By packing your veggies, fruits, and companion proteins the night before, you'll be armed for work, that weekend outing, or a plane trip. The cash value of my food skyrockets when I am the envy of the surrounding passengers sitting on a grounded plane on a runway for hours.

• Grocery shopping can be an adventure. Be creative as you walk through the fruit and veggie section. Are there veggies you don't recognize? Investigate. You may discover some great Hard Chews you've never had before. Venture toward the dairy section to find some new companion proteins. Soy cheese and tofu, as well as some interesting low-fat cheeses, come in a variety of flavors: jalapeno, dill, or peppercorn.

• Keep your refrigerator and cupboard stocked with snacks and ingredients for your favorite meals. You can't be on the program if you don't have the food. And again, be creative. Try some new spices when you have the time. Check the list of recommended cookbooks on pages 189–90. One or two interesting veggies recipes can be just the ticket to add spark to your menu.

• Invest in an insulated food bag. They are lightweight, inexpensive, and easily available. These handy bags are not only a practical way to carry your food with you where you go but they also become symbols of the new place food has in your life, helping you never to leave home without it.

• Write yourself reminders to prepare your food and supplements. It takes a while to trade one style of eating for another.

Leave Post-it notes on your mirror, your briefcase, on top of your bureau, wherever you are most likely to see them. Soon you'll be doing all this planning in your head but until the program is second nature, remind yourself.

• Embrace the idea that you have the power to nurture yourself, choose balance, and better your health. The joie de vivre will surely follow.

ADELE'S RECOMMENDED COOKBOOKS

The Soy Zone, Barry Sears, Ph.D. (New York: Regan Books, HarperCollins, 2001).

• This book has good ideas for innovative ways to use soy to introduce an interesting new dimension to eating. Its drawback is that it uses blocks of measurement in the Zone manner, which is cumbersome. Readers should not use those ways to measure their amounts. Therefore, format is confusing to understand, difficult to relate to, and hard to look at. If readers can go directly to the heart of the recipe they will have really good-tasting alternatives for meals.

The Ultimate Low-Carb Diet Cookbook, Donna Pliner Rodnitzky (New York: Prima Publishing, Random House, Inc., 2001).

• Varied and useful recipes range from dips and salads to main dish offerings for fish, poultry, tofu, and meat. Easy-to-make, interesting recipes with simple instructions.

• The author also offers dessert recipes that can be used in self-defense at parties or on special occasions *only*. Otherwise these desserts are not recommended. The drawback is that Sugar Babies may take the dessert recipes as an invitation to plunge in, which while low to moderate in carbohydrates, can keep the sweet connection going and can easily be abused by eating too much too often.

The Carbohydrate Addict's Cookbook, Richard F. Heller, Rachael F. Heller, et al. (New York: J. Wiley, 2001).

• Good all-around cookbook, simple to follow.

Low-Carb Cookbook, Fran McCullough (New York: Hyperion, 1997).

• Very attractive book with interesting and slightly exotic recipes for entrees and vegetables. Ignore the desserts unless you're having company; they are much too high in fat.

Vegetables, James Peterson (New York: William Morrow and Company, Inc., 1998).

• Nice all-round vegetable recipes with an attractive layout. You need to be selective here. Don't give yourself permission to indulge in the high-end carbs. Check the Giant Food List to decide.

Chez Panisse Vegetables, Alice Waters (New York: HarperCollins, 1996).

• Excellent vegetable ideas with attractive illustrations. Not all recipes are suitable. You need to use discretion and check the Giant Food List.

Cookbooks abound with many wonderful recipes for complex carbohydrates. Go to the bookstore and have fun browsing the shelves to find ideas on how to make delicious lentil pilaf or exotic brown rice medley. You will be surprised at how little you miss that nightly serving of mashed potatoes, if at all.

And while you are browsing, look through the vegetable cookbooks. Yes, there are books featuring vegetables, wonderful books written in answer to the desire of so many of us to eat in a healthy way. If your most familiar encounter with veggies is canned peas and carrots, get ready for a new taste sensation.

Vegetarian books offer some exciting and different recipes, but do be selective. The nature of vegetarian eating is reliant on an abundance of complex carbohydrates as the mainstay of the diet. Those of us with the Metabolic Mix-Up will not fare well unless we are extra careful about the recipes chosen. Of course recipes that feature tofu may be fine. If a high complex carbohydrate recipe catches your eye, refer to the Giant Food List to select foods from pure-power or middle-road categories. And remember to use small portions (fist size) of carbohydrates and partner them with protein and lots of vegetables.

BEING A PEERLESS PEER

We're never too old to be affected by those around us. Hard as we might try, how people treat us, what they think of us, and how they make us feel can disrupt our lives and distract us. I always find it interesting how whenever we decide to make a change in our lives, particularly a positive, life-altering change like the Midlife Miracle Diet, it triggers strong emotions in *other* people—especially those we are closest to. Why is this? Basically, change scares people even when it's a good one. When you begin to take positive steps to take care of yourself, others may feel guilty, knowing they should be doing the same. Your spouse or best friend or boss might react, fearing you are rocking the proverbial boat. Perhaps your wife loses her drinking partner or your husband might feel threatened when you stop joining him for dessert every evening. Even though some of those around you could react strongly and negatively to your new way of eating, they don't have to impact on you. It is really important that you don't get lost in their issues or reactions. This is about you. For you. Don't be surprised if you have trouble keeping your commitment to your new way of eating when people you love and respect are pressuring you to forget it for the evening or are criticizing you for being too uptight about your new food choices. Their seductive voices can pressure you to have what they have, making you feel as though your choice will affect their enjoyment. Be prepared to stay committed. We still want to be part of the group—a peerless peer.

If you feel confident and don't look bereft or defensive, and you are sure that what you are doing is good for you, then others will not only believe in you, they may also follow you. They will soon understand that no one is forcing you to eat well, that you are choosing to receive the rewards that following the four steps can bring, and that there is tremendous power in such a step. Reassure them calmly that you love what you are doing and explain that this is a choice you've made and you'd like their support. They may be able to hear you and stop criticizing and pressuring you to go off your diet. But if they cannot support you, don't try to convince them, and don't expect their cooperation. What an ideal world this would be if the people we care about were always supportive of the positive choices we make. But we all know this is not always the case, especially with family members. The rules have been played for years and changing the dynamics may be hard to do. Just encourage them to enjoy their foods and not worry about you, and use your energy for yourself. You'll feel better moving through your life, living it and enjoying your health the way you were meant to be.

CHAPTER 11

"Can I Ever Eat Bread Again?" and Other Questions

In my heart, anyone who reads this book is a client of mine—a client I care about. So, whether you've walked through my office door in New York City, or into your local bookstore and picked up *The Carb-Careful Solution,* I want to answer all your questions—and I know you have them! Some questions have been asked so often that I've been keeping a list of them over the years: questions the people I see in my private practice have asked, as well as questions friends and family members have asked, everything from traveling in different time zones to managing foods at the office to whether they will always have the Metabolic Mix-Up.

In the Questions and Answers you have a further opportunity to observe the program in action as they highlight both the trouble spots and their solutions, allowing you to anticipate potential challenges as you embark on the Carb-Careful Solution.

1. Am I going to have this Metabolic Mix-Up forever?
Possibly so. As some people lose weight they also lose their reactiveness to carbohydrates. But if you're like me and millions of other people sensitive to carbohydrates, you will continue to be somewhat vulnerable to your chemistry and always be on the

lookout for it to rear its powerful head. The degree to which your genes play a role in your mix-up will decide just how much attention you will have to pay to your reactiveness. Most important, even if you have the genes, you don't have to express them. By stabilizing your chemistry, you can change your reactions to the foods you eat. And although you may always have a body chemistry that is challenged by insulin resistance, the program enables you to keep the mix-up at bay and live life to the fullest.

2. How will I know that I fit the profile?

You should suspect that you have the Metabolic Mix-Up if your weight has been bouncing around your middle for your entire life, and if type 2 diabetes or stubborn high blood pressure runs in your family. Review the questionnaires and checklists in Chapter Three, using them as a further guide. You should also consult your health-care practitioner and make sure you receive the appropriate tests, including checking your homocysteine levels, triglycerides, HDL and LDL, blood pressure, glucose tolerance, and insulin levels.

3. I thought that fat-burner supplements were only for losing weight? How do they change my insulin resistance?

Of course these powerful supplements help you look better by burning fat, but they also help decrease your insulin resistance. The more fat deposits on your body, the more insulin resistant your body is. It's a catch-22. The more resistant your cells, the more insulin is produced. And the more hyperinsulinemic you are, the more your body is triggered into laying down fat. Know that you will also help to recondition your cells to become more able to utilize the insulin by incorporating all the steps to help you lose weight and reduce fat.

4. Does the Carb-Careful Solution mean I can never eat bread again?

It depends on you. Bread, after all, is a trigger carb, but depending on how much you exercise and what supplements you take and what combinations you create, you should be able to reintroduce and enjoy bread in moderation. But observe your reactions. Remember that exercising will help your body be more receptive while supplements can ease the passage of insulin into the cells. Your responses may vary, depending on how much you exercise and what supplements you take. Also, if you couple bread with a good fat such as olive oil, you cut its glycemic effect. But keep in mind that by becoming Carb-Careful you will miss the bread less and less. It may be hard to imagine, but it's true.

5. I know I look and feel better when I exercise, but aren't there other important benefits?
Exercising not only increases your endurance (stamina) but it also helps to build denser bones and raises HDL (good cholesterol) while it lowers high blood pressure and cardiovascular risk. Exercise also vastly improves your body composition by increasing the ratio of muscle mass to body mass. Together these factors tame your Metabolic Mix-Up and make you a leading candidate for vibrant health.

6. I'm a person with the perfect profile for the Metabolic Mix-Up. If body composition is a measure of how vital our health can be, then I fail miserably. I watch the fat build and ebb on my body on an almost daily basis. How can I really get rid of the fat while gaining muscle?
The Carb-Careful Solution's four steps will lead you to improve your body composition. Reconnect with:
  Basic Balance
  Carb Careful
  Supplement Solution
  Exercise Euphoria

7. What do I do when I go to a restaurant?
Choose wisely and make life easy for yourself by trying to eat at restaurants that can let you be reasonable. Try to dine on the early side. Arrival of courses can come only after you have placed

your order and the chef has time to cook it. You may not see your food for forty-five minutes to an hour or longer, depending on how busy the restaurant is and how quickly you order.

Remember to eat according to the reasonable range guides (for reasonable amounts see pages 63–64) and don't get so distracted by the attractive offerings that you forget to ask how the dish is prepared. If you include starches and sugars, remember to add a companion protein. I avoid Japanese restaurants, for example, because the white rice in sushi is not worth the damage it does. Of course if you are a sushi fanatic, then just ask for less rice and skip the sugar-laden ginger dressing that usually accompanies the salads offered in Japanese restaurants. The soy sauce winds up covering my waist. But if you have sashimi and sidestep the rice, you can still indulge your taste buds. The more you get to know your body and its reactions to certain foods, the easier it will become to choose restaurants where you can enjoy yourself without upsetting your balance and good blood sugar.

8. How will I ever live without my desserts?

This sounds like a question for someone whose chemistry is still at play. Are you having trouble with Carb-Careful and have you not yet locked your blood sugar balance into place? Chocolate fudge sundaes should not be eaten nightly by anyone. This type of sugar-loaded food will wreak havoc for anyone long-term. Save that hot fudge sundae for a special occasion, and divert yourself with a plate of blueberries and half-and-half—a sumptuous taste that could fill the void. If you absolutely must have your decadent dessert, make it important, have as little as possible to make you happy, and check your journal to see why your blood sugar is whispering sweet nothings in your ear.

9. Should I be concerned about processed foods?

There's been much discussion over the years about the lack of nutritional content and use of preservatives being possibly carcinogenic. But processed foods can be harmful to your health in other ways. They are loaded with hidden carbohydrates and sodium, and they are devoid of fiber, leaving room to need lots of food to fill you up. All of these factors make them highly re-active trigger foods for those of us with the Metabolic Mix-Up.

10. Should I make a commitment to eliminating all fat from my diet?

No. There is good fat and bad fat. *Good* fats supply the essential fatty acids that are contained in monounsaturated (olives, olive oil, avocado, almonds, pistachios, and macademia nuts) and un-saturated fats (those found in fish that supply us with omega-3 oils). *Bad* fat, the kind that clogs our arteries and contributes to such conditions as stroke, is called saturated fat. This bad fat comes from animal products and saturated vegetable oils. The es-sential fatty acids (EFAs) are absolutely critical for allover body metabolism and functioning. But it is the ratio of omega-3 fatty acids and monounsaturated fat to saturated fat that is important. Most Americans eat foods that have too much saturated fat, cre-ating a ratio that is too low in essential fatty acids. If you choose meats and milk products more often than salmon and almonds, it is vital that you take your EFAs in supplement form. See Chap-ter Seven for guidance.

11. If I am eating a late dinner, should I eat a late lunch?

Your on-time lunch will be your best friend. This may sound difficult to do at this point when you're just getting started, but one of the keys to the program is to create a rhythm in keeping with your body. Life does happen and occasionally you can't be able to stay on schedule, just be sure to eat as soon as you can. If you can't eat lunch by 1:00 P.M., try to maintain your snacks. And if you know dinner is going to be late, be sure to keep all other snacks in place. Have an extra snack in the afternoon, adding a companion protein to bolster your balance.

12. Why can't I skip breakfast if I get up late on a weekend?

For the same reason you should not eat a late lunch just to ac-commodate eating a late dinner, it's also important not to skip breakfast even if you get up late. Your body works on a circadian rhythm, and it needs to be treated as regularly as possible. If five days a week it is accustomed to awakening early and receiving breakfast at 7:30 A.M., then that's what it will be missing. So play catch up and deliver the food as soon as you wake up to get into balance, especially since Metabolic Mix-Up people are usually extremely sensitive. Even a late-wake-up breakfast at 9 or 10 A.M. requires lunch by 1 P.M.

13. I overate last night, so to compensate, I skipped the protein with breakfast the next morning. Is this okay?
Sorry! First, don't stress about last night's indulgences, you're human. But don't perpetuate the problem by cutting back on breakfast. That is actually an ingrained part of the diet culture we live in and nothing could be less helpful, physically as well as mentally. The surest way to start a binge is to withhold food from yourself by skipping breakfast. This is usually either a punishment for last night's splurge or a misguided afterthought to make up for the food indulgence. Just begin the day as usual, with the right combination, and remember: Every day is a new beginning with no time for any regrets for yesterday. Carpe diem!

14. Help! I'm beginning to crave my trigger food! What do I do?
First, don't worry! This usually happens to all of us at one time or another. The first step is to examine your food journal to see what you've been doing. What's going on? Have you been following the steps? Or maybe you forgot an afternoon snack a few days ago, or perhaps opted for something a little racier? This is where yesterday's eating will impact on today. Just keep working the steps and within one or two days, you'll be in balance again.

But if this is not the case and you've been faithful to the diet, then look a little closer at other things going on in your life. How is your stress level? Are you taking your supplements? Do you need to reduce or increase them? Has work become more difficult? Is your relationship with your family, friends, and your spouse or partner tense? Are you using foods instead of feeling your feelings? If so, then your recent cravings have more to do with your life than your body. Start by feeling your feelings and keep working the steps. Balance is right around the corner.

15. How do I modify my diet if I'm going on a plane in different time zones?

BYOS: Bring your own snacks! And if it's a morning flight, make sure you eat breakfast before boarding. If you have waited to have one of an airline's breakfast special, then you are eating too late. Plus, what if the plane is delayed? It's always important to start your trip off with balanced blood sugar. If it's an afternoon or evening flight, then really try to have whatever main meal is the last one before takeoff at your home or office, particularly if it's a long flight. And again, *bring your own snacks.*

A *perk:* You'll find that if you're going to Europe or some other distant time zone, your jet lag will be much less severe if you stabilize your blood sugar. You automatically give yourself a boost in energy and help stabilize your hormones. I also suggest bringing a large bottle of water to keep yourself hydrated. And don't start eating in the airport. Those candy bars that are calling your name will only make you pay later, depleting your good balance and energy and perhaps even ruining your trip. Besides, if you are going to do something to upset your chemistry, isn't it better to wait until you arrive to eat something extraordinary in a wonderful restaurant?

NOTE: If you're particularly concerned about how to handle traveling abroad and staying on the Carb-Careful Solution, consult Chapter Ten, where I deal with this question in depth.

16. I have bad PMS. Will being on the Carb-Careful Solution help it?

Yes. It's just another fringe benefit that you get from being on the diet. Reduced bloating and moodiness should certainly be expected on the program. You can also look for a decrease in water retention when you're following the steps. If you're controlling insulin behavior, then you are impacting the endocrine system, the overall system that regulates your hormones. By eating foods that don't challenge your Metabolic Mix-Up, you allow all systems to operate in a more balanced and harmonious state.

17. Can I eat foods not on the Giant Food List?

As you know, my list is really extensive, so if it's not on it, it probably means it should be regulated. It's important to remember that the Carb-Careful Solution is not a temporary quick-fix scheme; it's a way of life. And once you're on it, you're going to enjoy the feelings of balance and energy so it will soon be a natural part of your life. Read over Chapter Nine for tips on bringing the program with you, wherever you are.

18. Can I do this program without vitamin supplements?

The supplements are designed to calm the Metabolic Mix-Up and work synergistically with the rest of the steps. Changing your eating style and increasing your exercise are effective, so it is your choice. I do know that without the supplements, you are shortchanging yourself. Also, remember that when you take your supplements you can reintroduce some of your carbs. Supplements give you more freedom to eat with ease.

I have tried to anticipate and answer the most common questions, but don't worry if I have not. Sometimes it's easy to get nervous when you're beginning a new way of life. I promise the pieces will fall into place. Have faith; the Carb-Careful Solution will change your chemistry and become the way you eat, naturally. You will develop a new lifestyle that will support you. If you're feeling even the least bit overwhelmed, take a deep breath, clear your mind, and review the four steps. The answers really are all here, and some of them you already know yourself since it was you who picked up this book in the first place.

A Final Note: Just One More Conversation

Please come in and take that chair over there. It's time to send you out into the world, but before I do that I would like to share a little private time with you.

During the time we have spent together I've shared many of my clients' stories. I've also told you about talking to your chemistry and how your body reacts to stress, to foods, and to the world around you. I've warned you about the insulin factor and the way food can affect your well-being.

But the question remains: Have I made an impression? Are you ready to leave this office and conquer the world? Are you ready to take charge of your health and change your life? Those are the questions that only you can answer. I can only take your hand and try to lead you in a direction. It is you who possess the power and will to change.

So before we say good-bye let me remind you of a few things. The focus of most diets is to lose weight; with the Carb-Careful Solution it's not the focus, but a wonderful by-product. Yes, I am concerned about the outside of you looking good, but I am much more concerned with reengineering the inside of you so that you can maintain the *new you* forever. I want you to become healthy and then stay that way, by reversing high blood pressure and preventing type 2 diabetes and heart disease—just a few of the more important life-threatening diseases that we are all at risk of developing as we age.

And with this reengineering comes additional benefits: You will look younger and your skin will glow. You will reverse the damaging effects of premature aging caused by your insulin resistance, the heart of your Metabolic Mix-Up. You will achieve chemical balance and gain the wonderful feeling that accompanies it.

Should I worry that you will not be able to stay on the program? Not a chance, because once you have started the program and walked the steps, you will see how natural it becomes. You will feel so much better physically and mentally that you'll never want to go back to your old ways. Detours are no problem either; they are just a part of the process. Just examine what's happened, review your journals, remember how you felt when you were following the steps, and the solution will be easy. "I'm back!" my client Robert said. "The diet is about eating right and making myself feel better. Why do I stay with it? I stay with it because now that I know what feeling good is, I can't stand the way I feel when I'm not walking the steps. I go on with my scheduling so I can go on with my life."

I've seen lives transformed by being on the Midlife Miracle Diet. Like Marilyn, who admitted that she would never have had the courage to start her great new job or the focus to even know she should go after getting it. Or Tyler, who finally started a sculpture class, a lifelong dream that he'd never told anyone about. By following the steps, you too can be part of the many people who take control of their chemistry and change the direction of their lives.

Well, the time to say good-bye has come. But is it really good-bye? No, not really because you have at your disposal the knowledge of the Carb-Careful Solution. And in that knowledge is not a good-bye, but a hello to a new beginning. As you leave the door of my office, another door will open and in that room is your new beginning filled with the joy of good health, a sense of good feelings, and the beginning of a new and prosperous life. Know that I carry you in my heart and hope that you reach the best you can possibly be.

APPENDIX 1:
SAMPLE JOURNAL ENTRIES

KATHERINE IS FEELING BETTER FAST

Katherine is a woman in her early fifties. She is a very active sales and marketing executive who travels extensively for her job, but she always manages to work in her exercise and eat well. Take a look at how well she did during this week in which she flew from New York to Chicago and then out to the West Coast.

Monday

5:30 red pepper and cottage cheese
7:30 kirby cucumber and tuna envelope
9:30 green beans
11:30 red cabbage
12:30 salad and grilled chicken and green beans
3:30 plum and soy cheese
6:30 celery
7:30 salad and grilled salmon

water: 10 glasses
2-mile walk

ADELE'S NOTE: She added the soy cheese with her morning snack because she woke early and her lunch was seven hours later—too long a span to go without eating.

Tuesday

6:00 red pepper and cottage cheese
8:00 green beans
10:30 fennel
12:00 celery
12:45 salad and tuna, green beans
3:45 green beans
6:45 salad and grilled chicken

water: 10 glasses
3-mile walk

ADELE'S NOTE: Katherine is doing great!

Wednesday

5:30 red pepper and cottage cheese
7:30 green beans and tuna envelope
9:30 fennel
11:30 celery
12:45 chef salad with egg white, green beans
3:45 plum and soy cheese
6:45 celery
7:30 salad and grilled mahimahi

water: 10 glasses
2-mile walk

ADELE'S NOTE: By the third day, she is clearly in Basic Balance.

Thursday

5:30 red pepper and cottage cheese
7:30 green beans
9:30 celery
11:30 kirby
1:00 chinese chicken salad with water chestnuts and bok choy
4:00 apple with a few almonds
7:00 salad and grilled veggies, burger with mustard

water: 10 glasses
3-mile walk

Friday

5:30 red pepper and cottage cheese
7:30 celery and peanut butter
9:30 green beans
11:30 kirby
1:00 grilled shrimp with peppers and onions in a tamarind sauce, radish on side
4:00 pear and soy cheese
7:00 salad, baked sole with asparagus

water: 10 glasses
2-mile walk

ADELE'S NOTE: By Friday, Katherine has achieved her goal: *better balance!*

Saturday

8:00 celery and peanut butter
10:00 green beans
12:00 celery
1:00 salad and lemon chicken

4:00 *apple and cottage cheese*
7:00 *spinach salad and grilled calamari*

water: 10 glasses
3-mile walk

Sunday

 8:00 *celery and peanut butter*
10:00 *green beans*
12:00 *green beans*
 1:00 *egg white omelet and grilled veggies*
 4:00 *apple and soy cheese*
 7:00 *salad and grilled swordfish*

water: 10 glasses
5-mile walk

ADELE'S NOTE: This client had a fabulous week. My only suggestion to her was to try to vary her snacks and dishes more. You
never want to feel bored with your foods, so consult your Giant
Food List and get familiar with the fabulous array of foods and
food combinations to keep your tastebuds interested!

HENRY IS GOING TO HAVE TROUBLE

A fiftyish man, who runs his own retail store. Though he's on his
feet all day, he has not yet been able to schedule exercise on a
regular basis. He's also had a more difficult time establishing
Basic Balance right away. Take a look how his week unfolded.

Monday

6:15 *chicken and bread*
8:00 *cucumber*

9:15 *cucumber*
1:00 *salmon, salad, cucumber, balsamic dressing, water*
3:00 *apple with cottage cheese*
5:30 *cucumber*
7:15 *tilapia, broccoli*

ADELE'S NOTE: It's no wonder that this client complained he felt tired. I explained to him that this was the result of the too-long stretch between his morning snacks and lunch.

Tuesday

6:15 *toast with nut butter*
8:30 *kirby cucumber*
10:00 *kirby cucumber*
12:30 *tomatoes, chicken, and mushroom omelette—at desk*
3:00 *apple and nuts*
5:30 *cake*
8:30 *grilled veggies and mussels*

ADELE'S NOTE: I was not surprised to hear that this client found himself interested in reading every offering on the dinner menu, which means that he was not in either basic or better balance by the end of the day. Adding a small quantity of protein with his last snack would have helped prevent any triggering at his very late dinner.

Wednesday

7:00 *toast with nut butter*
9:00 *carrot*
10:30 *celery*
12:30 *gazpacho, salad, chicken breast sandwich*
3:00 *celery*
5:00 *celery*
7:30 *apple*
9:00 *salad, ½ sandwich, potato salad*

ADELE'S NOTE: He is starting to wander into more carbs because of his late dinner and not adding a Hard Chew lunch. Once again, he had failed to add a protein to his last snack, which would have fortified his balance.

Thursday

7:00 rye toast with nut butter
8:30 cake
10:00 cake
12:30 salad with tuna, radish, carrots
3:00 cake
5–6:00 pretzels
6:00 apple
8:00 pizza, big salad, wine, pretzels, crackers to 2 A.M.

ADELE'S NOTE: He was feeling happy (probably because of eating all his favorite foods), but tired—for the same reason: He ate too many Lower Rung foods, which may feed the soul but they also lower the blood sugar!

Friday

7:00 rye toast with nut butter
8:30 cake
10:00 cake
12:30 steamed chicken with broccoli and rice, 2 dumplings
8:00 3 steamed dumplings

ADELE'S NOTE: We can be sure that he awakened in low blood sugar, compliments of his too-rich dinner the night before. The loss of his *better balance* puts him in the position of looking for trouble from the very beginning of the day.

Saturday

7:30 bread with tuna
12:30 grilled veggies, salad
8:00 steak, french fries, salad

ADELE'S NOTE: Given his dinner choice on Saturday, he is clearly longing for high-fat food and starchy foods—his body is literally craving those foods, a sure sign that his Metabolic Mix-Up has moved back in. He'll never know what he's missing.

Sunday

11:00 bread and cheese
12:30 apple
1:30 bag of pretzels
3:00 cake
4:30 salad, turkey burger on roll, pasta salad, zucchini
8:00 cake and two cookies

ADELE'S NOTE: He said he didn't feel like dinner, but he knew he had to eat it anyway. And he should have eaten lunch as well! Remember, skipping meals is never a good idea! If he'd had either or both meals, the cookies and cake may never have left the bakery! He didn't let himself get into *better balance*.

SUSAN OWNS THIS PROGRAM!

Susan is a busy mother of three.

Monday

7:30 rye crackers and cottage cheese
9:30 apple and slice of low-fat cheddar cheese
11:00 string beans

1:10 lemon chicken, chopped salad with chunks of red cabbage, and
      French string beans
4:00 plum
6:30 steamed shrimp and broccoli

water: 2 1-liter bottles of water
exercise: brief walk

ADELE'S NOTE: Susan enjoyed this toned-down dinner. It was a wise idea to balance the larger than usual lunch.

Tuesday

 7:30 egg-white veggie omelet
10:00 celery stalk
12:15 inside of tuna sandwich and celery
 2:00 blueberries and a little cottage cheese
 5:00 cauliflower chunks
 7:30 veal chop, spinach, and zucchini

water: 2 1-liter bottles
exercise: none

ADELE'S NOTE: Susan wisely moved up her afternoon snack to an earlier time to satisfy her needs created by a lunch (she got caught doing errands and ate while driving!) that was less than satisfying.

Wednesday

 8:00 peanut butter in celery chunks
10:00 red cabbage
12:00 pear and sliced turkey breast
 1:00 tuna, chopped lettuce, and veggies
 4:15 string beans
 7:00 kirby cucumber and 2 shrimp

8:30 chicken and ½ yam and stir-fry broccoli; mixed raspberries
     and blueberries for dessert

water: 2 1-liter bottles
exercise: yoga class

ADELE'S NOTE: Susan really managed well. By adding protein to her second afternoon snack, she helped to fortify her blood sugar in anticipation of a late dinner. Having the fruit as dessert helped to prevent a dip into her husband's dessert.

Thursday

8:00 cottage cheese and leftover grilled veggies
10:30 apple and low-fat cheddar
12:00 discreet chef salad
3:00 apple and a thin layer of peanut butter
6:00 mixed crunchy veggies
7:00 red snapper, asparagus, and lentil salad

water: 3 1-liter bottles
exercise: long, 3-mile walk with a friend

ADELE'S NOTE: She continues to use her information very well.

Friday

7:45 toast and salmon
9:30 celery
11:00 pear and turkey
12:30 chicken salad, tomatoes, lettuce, and radishes
4:00 plum and almonds
6:30 string beans with a side teaspoon of peanut butter
8:45 strip steak, spinach, salad, and yam

water: 2 1-liter bottles
exercise: none

ADELE'S NOTE: Her chemistry is more cooperative than some; the occasional slice of bread at breakfast doesn't seem to be a problem. However, she would probably feel better and more energetic if she waited a night before including a starchy carb in her dinner—especially before the weekend.

Saturday

10:00 rye bread, scrambled eggs with peppers, tomatoes, and
        onions
12:15 Cobb salad
2:30 broccoli
5:00 apple with low-fat cheese
7:00 2 sparkling water and lemon, Cosmopolitan, veal marsala,
        mixed vegetables, and rice

water: 1 1-liter bottle
exercise: family bike ride

ADELE'S NOTE: Late wake-up following several nights of carbohydrates probably invited that Cosmopolitan when she and her husband went out to eat. An unmixed drink would be less challenging than the sweet cocktail, which went on to design the rest of Susan's menu.

Sunday

9:30 tofu and grilled veggies
11:30 fennel
12:30 roast chicken, salad, and asparagus
2:30 plum and cottage cheese
4:30 blueberries and half-and-half
6:00 pork chop and zucchini, broccoli, and cucumbers with gua-
        camole

water: 3 1-liter bottles
exercise: none

ADELE'S NOTE: Susan had a difficult day. But she did know that she had to be extremely careful because of Saturday night, so she kept her timing tighter than usual and added some higher fat foods to satisfy her taste buds. Susan realized that this would be the best way to offset the night before, making sure she reestablished her *better balance* when she chose to drink.

APPENDIX 2:
BLANK FOOD JOURNAL

Date	/	/	/	/	/	/	/
Day	Monday	Tuesday	Wednesday	Thursday	Friday	Saturday	Sunday
Breakfast	Time:	Time:	Time:	Time:	Time:	Time:	Time:
Snack	Time:	Time:	Time:	Time:	Time:	Time:	Time:
Snack	Time:	Time:	Time:	Time:	Time:	Time:	Time:
Lunch	Time:	Time:	Time:	Time:	Time:	Time:	Time:
Snack	Time:	Time:	Time:	Time:	Time:	Time:	Time:
Snack	Time:	Time:	Time:	Time:	Time:	Time:	Time:
Dinner	Time:	Time:	Time:	Time:	Time:	Time:	Time:
Comments							

FOR FURTHER READING

It has been my absolute pleasure to witness my many clients not only achieve better health but also, and more important, change their destiny through the Carb-Careful Solution. Observing these life-altering changes in the clinical setting has made me ever so grateful, and I wanted to share with you a brief sampling of the large body of scientific research where you too can see how and why the program works.

Anderson R. "Chromium in the Prevention and Control of Diabetes," *Diabetes and Metabolism* (Paris). 2000;26(1):22–27.

Bland, J.S. "New Functional Medicine Paradigm: Health Problems Associated with Dysfunctional Intercellular Communication," *International Journal of Integrative Medicine,* Jul/Aug 1999; 1(4): 11–16.

———. "Functional Medicine Approach to Managing Syndrome X and Type 2 Diabetes," *International Journal of Integrative Medicine,* Nov/Dec 1999; 1(6): 39–45.

——— and S.H. Benum. *Genetic Nutrioneering: How You Can Modify Inherited Traits and Live a Longer, Healthier Life.* Los Angeles: Keats, 1999.

Faure, P., et al. "Vitamin E Improves the Free Radical Defense

System Potential and Insulin Sensitivity of Rats Fed High Fructose Diets," *Journal of Nutrition,* 1997; 127:103–7.

Foster, D.W. "Insulin Resistance—a Secret Killer?" *New England Journal of Medicine,* 1989; 320 (11): 733–34.

French, R.J., and P.J.H. Jones. "Role of Vanadium in Nutrition: Metabolism, Essentiality and Dietary Considerations," *Life Sciences,* 1992; 52:339–46.

Halberstam, M. et al. "Oral Vanadyl Sulfate Improves Insulin Sensitivity in NIDDM but Not in Obese Nondiabetic Subjects," *Diabetes,* 1996; 45:659–66.

Kubota, N., et al. "PPARy Mediates High-Fat Diet-Induced Adipocyte Hypertrophy and Insulin Resistance," *Molecular Cell,* 1994: 597–609.

Liu, S., et al. "A Prospective Study of Dietary Glycemic Load, Carbohydrate Intake, and Risk of Coronary Heart Disease in US Women," *American Journal of Clinical Nutrition,* 2000; 71: 1455–461.

MacDonald, H.S. "Conjugated Linolenic Acid and Disease Prevention: A Review of Current Knowledge," *Journal of American College of Nutrition,* 2000; 19(2):111S–18S.

Mooy, J.M. "Major Stressful Life Events in Relation to Prevalence of Undetected Type 2 Diabetes—The Hoorn Study," *Diabetes Care,* February 2000.

Preuss, H.G. "Effects of Glucose/Insulin Perturbations on Aging and Chronic Disorders of Aging," *Journal of American College of Nutrition,* 1997; 16(5):397–403.

Reaven, G. *Syndrome X: Overcoming the Silent Killer That Can Give You a Heart Attack.* New York: Simon & Schuster, 1990.

Roberts, K., et al. "Syndrome X: Medical Nutritional Therapy," *Nutrition Review,* 2000; 58(5):154–60.

Rudich, A., et al. "Lipoic Acid Protects Against Oxidative Stress Induced Impairment in Insulin Stimulation of Protein Kinase B and Glucose Transport in 3T30L1 Adipocytes," *Diabetologia,* 1999;42:949–57.

Wahli, W., et al. "Fatty Acids, Eicosanoids, and Hypolipidemic Agents Regulate Gene Expression Through Direct Binding to

Perxisome Proliferator-Activated Receptors," *Lipoxygenases and Their Metabolites.* New York: Plenum Press, 1999.

Zhang, H., et al. "A High Biotin Diet Improves the Impaired Glucose Tolerance of Long-term Spontaneously Hyperglycemic Rats with Non-Insulin Dependent Diabetes Mellitus," *Journal of Nutrition Science Vitaminol,* 1996; 42: 517–26.

INDEX

Page numbers in *italics* refer to illustrations.

Adele Puhn would like to hear from you.
Please share your experiences with *The Carb-Careful Solution*
by contacting me at one of the following Web sites:

adelepuhn.com

or

midlifemiraclediet.com

or

5daymiraclediet.com

Adele is available for lectures, seminars, and workshops based
on this book or her previous works.
Details will be sent upon request.

FOR THE BEST IN PAPERBACKS, LOOK FOR THE

In every corner of the world, on every subject under the sun, Penguin represents quality and variety—the very best in publishing today.

For complete information about books available from Penguin—including Penguin Classics, Penguin Compass, and Puffins—and how to order them, write to us at the appropriate address below. Please note that for copyright reasons the selection of books varies from country to country.

In the United States: Please write to *Penguin Group (USA), P.O. Box 12289 Dept. B, Newark, New Jersey 07101-5289* or call *1-800-788-6262.*

In the United Kingdom: Please write to *Dept. EP, Penguin Books Ltd, Bath Road, Harmondsworth, West Drayton, Middlesex UB7 0DA.*

In Canada: Please write to *Penguin Books Canada Ltd, 10 Alcorn Avenue, Suite 300, Toronto, Ontario M4V 3B2.*

In Australia: Please write to *Penguin Books Australia Ltd, P.O. Box 257, Ringwood, Victoria 3134.*

In New Zealand: Please write to *Penguin Books (NZ) Ltd, Private Bag 102902, North Shore Mail Centre, Auckland 10.*

In India: Please write to *Penguin Books India Pvt Ltd, 11 Panchsheel Shopping Centre, Panchsheel Park, New Delhi 110 017.*

In the Netherlands: Please write to *Penguin Books Netherlands bv, Postbus 3507, NL-1001 AH Amsterdam.*

In Germany: Please write to *Penguin Books Deutschland GmbH, Metzlerstrasse 26, 60594 Frankfurt am Main.*

In Spain: Please write to *Penguin Books S. A., Bravo Murillo 19, 1° B, 28015 Madrid.*

In Italy: Please write to *Penguin Italia s.r.l., Via Benedetto Croce 2, 20094 Corsico, Milano.*

In France: Please write to *Penguin France, Le Carré Wilson, 62 rue Benjamin Baillaud, 31500 Toulouse.*

In Japan: Please write to *Penguin Books Japan Ltd, Kaneko Building, 2-3-25 Koraku, Bunkyo-Ku, Tokyo 112.*

In South Africa: Please write to *Penguin Books South Africa (Pty) Ltd, Private Bag X14, Parkview, 2122 Johannesburg.*